SIMPSON AND SYME
OF EDINBURGH

Made and Printed in Great Britain

EDINBURGH IN 1824
Syme was born at 56 Princes Street, a house at the East End.
St John's Church is in the foreground.

Frontispiece

SIMPSON AND SYME OF EDINBURGH

BY

JOHN A. SHEPHERD

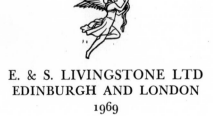

E. & S. LIVINGSTONE LTD
EDINBURGH AND LONDON
1969

TO
ALICE AND THE CHILDREN

Preface

Two remarkable Edinburgh doctors died a hundred years ago, James Syme and James Simpson. One was a surgeon and the other an obstetrician but both exerted great influence beyond their specialties. The range of their interests was such that from the study of their careers it is possible to bring to life the astonishing period of discovery and advance of medical science in the middle of the nineteenth century. In character these men were so different that a clash of their personalities was inevitable.

It has been my main objective to put their medical achievements into perspective but I have also gone quite deeply into the social and domestic background of their lives. Some may consider that an account of the jealousies, quarrels and intrigues, so characteristic of professional life in the Victorian Age, is irrelevant and that in retrospect these tensions and trials may seem petty, trivial and best forgotten. But this was a part of their lives and cannot be ignored if actions and characters are to be understood. Human nature does not change and in this story there may be lessons for us today, whether we are in medical, academic, political or any other walks of life.

Of the two protagonists Simpson established for himself a place in medical history from which he can never be dislodged. Syme is less well remembered but he was great in his time. Simpson's contributions are more memorable and more spectacular; Syme's work is of much significance especially when viewed against the state of contemporary surgical practice.

Simpson has never ceased to attract the interest of the medical historian, and indeed the lay public, because of his rise to international fame from a humble origin, his unique personality and, in particular, his discovery of the use of chloroform. There are at least three full biographies and his work and character have been analysed over the years in innumerable articles and orations. When he died his family saw it as their duty to find a biographer who would compile a memoir to meet with their approval and provide a fitting tribute. Such was the custom in the Victorian Age on the death of anyone of eminence—real or supposed. A friend, Dr Alexander Wood, was approached but he did not accept the task. The choice fell on the Reverend John Duns (1818–1903) Professor of Natural Science in New College, the training school of the Free Church created at the time of the Disruption. He had little eminence as a scientist and was not well fitted to assess Simpson's medical work. His primary interest was in Simpson's religious beliefs and if perhaps he overstressed this aspect this was in an accepted tradition for such a memoir. Duns' account is lengthy for he had known Simpson intimately in his last years and he had free access to all his papers. In parts it is tedious, sermonising and ill-arranged, but there is so much information that it is an essential source-book. Published in 1873, soon after Simpson's death, it is silent on many of the controversies in which he was involved. When it was reviewed it was said to show 'a bias and a one-sidedness which completely pervert the lessons to be derived from Simpson's life!' In particular Duns' elaboration on the alleged religious 'conversion' of Simpson in his later years was deplored. This life and a series of sanctimonious tracts which appeared later did much to create a false image.

In 1897, on the fiftieth anniversary of Simpson's discovery of the use of chloroform, a second biography was published by Henry Laing Gordon (1865–1947). This is a concise and uncritical record with emphasis on Simpson's contribution to anaesthesia. In general it is a synopsis of Duns' larger volume and adds little that is new. Gordon was an Edinburgh graduate who practised in London for some years as a neurologist. He became a restless traveller abroad until in time he settled in Kenya, to achieve some reputation as an authority on sociological problems in Africa.

Almost simultaneously, a third biography was written by Simpson's youngest daughter Eve. This also is brief but eminently readable for it gives an intimate picture of a much loved father. Eve Simpson was at pains to discount Duns' emphasis on the religious beliefs of his subject and her copy of his biography survives, heavily blue-pencilled over the passages to which she took exception.

In 1935 there appeared a novel entitled *Jamie Simpson*, written by Laurence Oliver, and dedicated to a descendant with the avowed intention of rescuing her grandfather from dull Victorian biographers. This is a fictional account of Simpson's early life. Most of the accepted anecdotes are woven into the story with some degree of accuracy but some imaginary and somewhat scurrilous details are introduced. In general there is a cheap dramatisation and an unforgiveable lack of taste.

For any subsequent writer Duns provides a wealth of material and his documentary sources can be checked, for they are almost all to be found in a large trunk of unsorted letters and papers bequeathed in 1946 to the Royal College of Surgeons of Edinburgh. Duns made rather a haphazard selection of this material and for obvious reasons did not use it all. There are many other collections which contain documents relating to Simpson, in fact the volume of material is almost embarrassing. I am well aware that I have not been able to tap every source of information but have listed those to which I have had access.

James Syme has not received so much attention and only one full biography is known. This was written by Robert Paterson (1814–1889) and published in 1874. Paterson, an intimate of both Syme and Simpson, was a well known Leith physician who became President of the Royal College of Physicians of Edinburgh. His memoir seems reliable and relatively unbiased; when it appeared it was accepted as a true picture of Syme. As such I have drawn on it heavily and it must be acknowledged as the only full account of his life. Many additional facts concerning Syme can be found in the numerous biographies of his son-in-law Joseph Lister and in the writings of John Brown and of other contemporaries. In more recent years, as compared with Simpson, there have been few articles on Syme but those I have traced are listed in the appendix. It is unfortunate that, whether by accident or design, remarkably few letters survive; Paterson had access to some of his correspondence but the originals cannot be traced.

Both Syme and Simpson were prolific writers and in their technical books and articles there are many details of their interests and their movements which aid the biographer. Both were almost obsessive correspondents to the medical and lay press and such letters are often illuminating. The medical journals of the nineteenth century are full of news of the doings of the better known physicians and surgeons of the day. If at times such items are mere gossip, or even verge on slander, they do provide clues of value and interest. Finally the obituaries in the medical journals are significant, for the Victorians were very frank and they did not always follow the injunction *de mortuis nil nisi bonum*.

I must thank the Wellcome Trust for a very generous grant towards the cost of publication of this book and for permission to use material from the Wellcome Library. The President and Council of the Royal College of Surgeons of Edinburgh have given me access to the remarkable collection of manuscripts and other items in their library and have permitted me to quote from this material. I am greatly indebted to the President of the Royal College of Surgeons of England, the President and Council of the Liverpool Medical Institution, the Edinburgh University Library and the R.A.M.C. Library, Millbank, for permission to use letters or other documents in their possession. The Editors of the *British Medical Journal* and the *Lancet* have allowed me to quote freely from these journals.

Chapman and Hall Ltd, Hamish Hamilton and John Murray have kindly permitted me to reprint short extracts from books which they have published and these are noted in the reference list.

In the list of Plates I have made due acknowledgement to the owners or custodians of the originals. Mr R. E. Hutchison and his staff in the Scottish National Portrait Gallery have been very helpful in tracing early portraits and photographs. Mr Alistair Gunn has let me see the comprehensive collection of Plates he made for his Simpson Memorial Lecture in 1967.

Miss Catherine Simpson, who has recently given to the Royal College of Surgeons of Edinburgh some important letters written by her grand-uncle, has from her knowledge of the Simpson family helped me bridge the past and the present.

Many librarians have given generous assistance and in particular I would thank Miss Dorothy Wardle, of the Royal College of Surgeons of Edinburgh; Mr. E. H. Cornelius, of the Royal College of Surgeons of England; Mr Charles Finlayson, Keeper of Manuscripts, of the Edinburgh University Library; and Mr Lee, of the Liverpool Medical Institution. Miss Ella Burt has once more prepared a typescript for me with great patience. To all concerned of E. and S. Livingstone Ltd I acknowledge the helpfulness and skill with which they have brought this work to completion. It is very appropriate that this book should be published in Edinburgh.

1969.   J. A. SHEPHERD.

Contents

List of Illustrations

xiii

CHAPTER 1

The Edinburgh Background

IN the second half of the eighteenth century the city of
Edinburgh spread from the crowded wind-swept ridge
between the Castle Rock and Holyrood to the new sites
lying north and south of the original mediaeval town. This
was the Augustan Age of Edinburgh, with an eminence in
art and literature acquired in a remarkably short period in
this the small capital of a relatively impoverished country.
The names of Ramsay, Raeburn, Adam, Hume, Robertson
and Mackenzie are only a few to represent those who contributed to this culture. In this period the population was
increased, until it stood at 67,300 in 1800. There was an influx
of Highlanders evicted from their lands after the Forty-five
Rebellion. There was a less readily absorbed entry of the
Irish. Most important of all the country lairds and the lesser
aristocracy of the Lowlands came into the capital. They
entered the professions rather than commerce and established a caste system and a tradition within which the arts
could flourish. While many of the more famous noble families
migrated to London and became absentee landlords, a few
remained and by their philanthropy and patronage exerted
great influence.

In James Craig, the age had a planner who exploited effectively the spacious site lying to the north of the Castle. Adam
and Playfair were architects with a magnificent flair for boldness in the lay-out of new streets and terraces and in the
planning of frontages and interior decoration.[1]

While the move from the Old to the New Town destroyed
some of the elegance of life in the eighteenth century, there
evolved a new society with less coarseness of speech, less
arrogance and rather less debauchery and drinking. Before

1

1800 at dinners, for example, as Cockburn records: 'healths and toasts were special torments: oppressions which cannot now be conceived. Every glass during dinner required to be dedicated to the health of someone. . . . Thus, where there were ten people there were ninety healths drunk.' But on such occasions conversation flowed around literature, art and philosophy. Debating societies flourished, but these were in private gatherings while public expression of ideas was almost non-existent. Political differences and personal animosities were the subject of vituperative anonymous pamphlets or letters. These weapons were adopted widely by the medical profession of the time.

To this cultured and civilised community came the impact of the French Revolution. At first the young, the idealistic and the poetic rejoiced and waxed enthusiastic, but Jacobinism or republican ideas were soon stamped upon by the Tory party, then holding most of the wealth and controlling all the public offices and institutions in the country. Any critic of the Tory party was suppressed, every political objector was held a Jacobin. There was a great fear, engendered by the overthrow of the French monarchy, of a rising of the masses. Rational or reforming opinions, such as were held by the Whigs, were expressed at great personal risk even by men who held high office in the legal profession or in the university. With the Whigs powerless the whole country was under oppression and Henry Dundas, Viscount Melville, was in Edinburgh regarded as a dictator. Cockburn described him as the Pharos of Scotland, 'who steered upon him was safe: who disregarded his light was wrecked. It was to his nod that every man owed what he had got, and looked for what he wished.' There was seldom a time of greater dominance by a political party but despite this there was intellectual freedom.

As a result of the French Revolution there was an influx of foreign refugees to Edinburgh and it brought new ideas particularly in science and in political economy. These visitors were delighted to find a cultured community of which the young at least offered a fertile soil for the implantation of fresh thought. Almost simultaneously Edinburgh became a centre of attraction for the English who until this time, with the exception of a literary coterie, knew little of Scotland

and indeed maintained an almost primitive distrust. This had been engendered in part by Prince Charles' abortive invasion of England in 1745 when London was in near panic as a straggling army of ill-equipped Highlanders got as far south as Derby. This awakening of interest in Scotland and the acceptance of Edinburgh as a centre of importance was enhanced by the writings of Walter Scott, which swept England and continental Europe.

The Tories dominated the national political scene until 1806 when they were ousted by the Whigs. Local affairs of the city were managed by the Town Council. This all-powerful self-elected body was described as 'omnipotent, corrupt, impenetrable; nothing was beyond its grasp; no variety of opinion disturbed its unanimity, for the pleasure of Dundas was the sole rule for every one of them.' While the political masters and the rich were treated with obeisance, the ordinary people were tyrannised by the Council. Not least of their monopolies was the right to elect the professors of the University. Local government, political institutions and the like were, in general, grossly defective. The principles of liberty, although held by many in theory, could not be enacted at the turn of the century. In consequence little was done for the poor, the law was excessively harsh and there was no improvement in the education of the common people. Only with increasing commercial prosperity, with the waning of revolutionary ideas and with the demise of the 'old hard aristocracy' did things improve. Thus Edinburgh, as London and other cities, was a contrast of wealth, culture and comfort alongside extreme poverty, debauchery and crime. The high 'lands' of the castle ridge, once the palaces of the noblest families, had become filthy, disease-ridden, overcrowded slums which scarcely had their equals in the whole of Europe.

The cultured society of Edinburgh reached its zenith about 1815 and after this date the older characters passed from the scene, many of the more brilliant young men went to London and the excitement of the Napoleonic Wars died. The intense literary and artistic output of the previous 50 years began to subside and the visitors from the Continent withdrew. With the downfall of the Tories in 1805 free speech was restored and reform was in the air. Even an early restoration of Tory rule did not damp this more liberal outlook. As the terror of the French Revolution receded the Tories could afford to be less hysterical and less oppressive.

The early nineteenth century was a unique period and men's thoughts were quickly turned into new channels. While the rapid advances of science were still to come to create industrial expansion to amass new wealth, and to improve communications and so to cause a great upheaval of life in town and country, the atmosphere was electric; to be born at the start of the century was to enter into a new inheritance. In the compact community of Edinburgh, in which already there were firmly established traditions of progressive thought and originality, no young man of reasonable ability and intelligence could fail to be infected by the urge for reform, for discovery and for invention. In particular the opportunities were great in the fields of science and medicine. University education was, in contrast to England, open to rich and poor alike. Thus it was that James Syme, born in 1799 of a relatively prosperous family occupying the higher social stratum of the city, did not have much advantage over James Simpson, born in 1811 of humble parents in an obscure Scottish country town. Nevertheless the differing social backgrounds had some repercussions in their respective careers.

To appreciate how these two men were educated and how they both attained such eminence and such dominant positions in medicine some of the history and contemporary background of the University, and in particular the Medical School, must be recounted.

The University was founded in 1582 but before this date, in 1506, James IV had granted the Barber Surgeons of Edinburgh a charter empowering them to decide by examination who might practise surgery in the burgh. From this charter there developed the Royal College of Surgeons of Edinburgh with rights to dissect the body of one executed criminal each year and so to encourage anatomical study. This was a somewhat limited arrangement for organised instruction but nevertheless it proved the beginning of medical teaching in Edinburgh. Rather surprisingly the College was also granted the monopoly of the sale of aqua vitae. This monopoly, unfortunately for the funds of the College, was not perpetuated.

4

While the teaching of anatomy and surgery was established at this early date it was not until 1681, with the foundation of the College of Physicians, that the teaching of medicine was organised. In 1685 two Professors of Medicine were appointed by the College to be associated with the University and one of them was Archibald Pitcairn (1652-1713). In 1692 Pitcairn went to Leyden as Professor of Medicine, language offering no difficulty as in all universities the teaching was in Latin. This appointment established a link between Edinburgh and Leyden which was to influence the rapid growth and increasing fame of the Edinburgh Medical School. John Monro (1670-1737) studied medicine at Leyden under Pitcairn and then became an army surgeon. He returned to his native country so impressed by the methods of teaching in Leyden (which had absorbed the best elements of Padua) that he was determined to introduce them to Edinburgh. To achieve this he sent his son Alexander to Leyden for his medical education, with the express intention of grooming him for the Chair of Anatomy in Edinburgh. This, the first of many examples of calculated nepotism in the creation of medical professors, was entirely successful. In 1720 Alexander Monro *primus* (1697-1767) became professor and not only did he establish the Edinburgh school firmly, but also he ensured the remarkable succession of three Monros, *primus, secundus* and *tertius*, who held the same chair in direct descent for a period of 126 years. Monro *primus* and his son Alexander Monro *secundus* (1733-1817) were great teachers and contributed equally to the advance of anatomy and to the development of the Medical School. Alexander Monro *tertius* (1773-1859) was perhaps rather less successful and it is said that the students delighted to cheer and shower him with peas when he solemnly ploughed through his grandfather's lecture notes and read 'when I was a student in Leyden in 1719'. This oft quoted story is probably apocryphal and tends to derogate Monro *tertius* who had many virtues but, holding his chair for so long, outlived his period. Amongst others Charles Darwin, during his short period of medical study in Edinburgh, was excessively bored by Monro's lectures. Monro *tertius* blocked the way for such able anatomists as the brothers John Bell (1763-1820) and Charles Bell (1774-1842) either of whom could have held the Chair with greater distinction than the ageing Monro. The uninspiring teaching of Monro's later period had much to do with the success of the extra-mural schools in Edinburgh, in which anatomy was taught so ably by men such as John Barclay (1758-1826) and Robert Knox (1791-1862). In many ways the extra-mural schools proved of great benefit, not least in that a total of 37 professors in the University began their careers as lecturers in these unofficial organisations. But it was inevitable that when the more brilliant extra-mural lecturers attracted students away from the University, that rivalries should ensue and that the University was weakened. Quarrels developed particularly over hospital appointments and induced some able individuals, particularly the surgeons, to leave Edinburgh. This was often of great advantage to the London schools.[2, 3, 4]

The teaching of surgery in the eighteenth century was closely linked with anatomy and not until 1831 was the University Chair of Surgery made separate from that of anatomy. James Russel (1755-1836) was however appointed to a University Chair of Clinical Surgery in 1803. The Infirmary Governors selected six surgeons to take charge of patients in their institution. The tenure of office was for five years and the appointments were given in rotation to Fellows of the College of Surgeons. While this was an improvement on an older system by which physicians and surgeons held office in turn for only a month, it had great disadvantages. A good teacher might be superseded after five years and replaced by a nonentity. There was no continuity, little likelihood of the maintenance of high standards and the system was discouraging to ambitious young men. Although Russel was Professor of Clinical Surgery for most of his career he had no beds and required to lecture on patients provided by his colleagues. It says much for his tact that in doing so he rarely incurred the enmity of his fellow surgeons.

The College of Surgeons, recognising the highly unsatisfactory state of affairs, tried to improve this in 1804 by appointing their own Professor of Surgery. Not surprisingly the Senate of the University was greatly displeased. The first College professor was John Thomson (1765-1846) who two

6

years later took up, and held simultaneously, the crown appointment of Professor of Military Surgery in the University. He relinquished both these posts when in 1831 he became the first to occupy the Chair of Pathology in Edinburgh. Robert Knox called Thomson 'the old chairmaker', not only in reference to his extraordinary versatility in holding three professorships, but also because of his manipulations of other appointments.

That there was a chair of military surgery before the creation of a chair of pure surgery was not entirely surprising. John Bell, distinguished not only for his surgical contributions but for his influence in establishing anatomy as a practical subject relating directly to surgery, had petitioned the government during the Napoleonic Wars to establish teaching in military surgery. He was aware of the poor training and the inefficiency of most of the army surgeons and he considered that the universities should correct this. Surgery after all, at that time, was largely concerned with the management of inflammations and wounds and a very large proportion of the doctors of the British Isles were in the army or navy. Thomson had no military experience except that, like Charles Bell and other civil surgeons, he had rushed to the scene of Waterloo to render assistance to the wounded and dying lying neglected after the battle. Thomson was succeeded by George Ballingal (1780-1855) whose military experience was rather more extensive and he held the Chair until 1855 when it was finally abolished (during the Crimean War when perhaps it was greatly needed!). There was always some doubt as to the true function and status of the Professor of Military Surgery. Although his class included a proportion of officers from the services he also taught students. Unlike the Professor of Clinical Surgery he at least had his own beds.

Although Edinburgh had a wealth of able surgical teachers the organisation up to 1831, when John Turner (1790-1836) was appointed Professor of Surgery, was confused and inadequate. James Syme when he became Professor of Clinical Surgery in 1833 found there was need for much reform.

In contrast to the somewhat erratic organisation of surgical teaching, which did not always enhance the reputation of the University, medical teaching by 1800 had a high reputation and this alone had much to do with the fame of Edinburgh as a centre attracting students, not only from the British Isles but from all over the world. William Cullen (1710-1790), James Gregory (1753-1821) and Andrew Duncan (1744-1828) were prominent amongst the physicians to whom such large numbers of students flocked. Chairs in the practice of medicine and in the institutes of medicine had been founded long before 1800. Closely linked with the teaching of medicine were the chairs in chemistry, in fact it was not unusual for professors to teach both subjects or to transfer from one chair to the other. Joseph Black (1728-1799) and Thomas Hope (1766-1844) were two notable professors of chemistry who had much more to do with the medical faculty than their successors today. Although in theory and practice medicine had advanced little over 200 years, at least it could be affirmed that the University taught the subject thoroughly and that the physicians of the time were men of great character and ability.

The third major branch of medicine, midwifery, was ill-developed in 1800. Although as early as 1726 a surgeon Gibson (?-1739) of Leith had persuaded the Town Council to appoint him as City Professor of Midwifery, he had no place in the Senate and he instructed midwives but not students. In 1756 Thomas Young (?-1783) at least taught students, but his few beds were in an attic in the Infirmary. The status of the obstetrician remained low and practice continued to be largely the prerogative of ill-trained midwives until Alexander Hamilton (1739-1802) became professor in 1780. He contributed greatly to the establishment of the subject as a reputable science and, in the manner of the time, brought up his son James to succeed him. Father and son created, partly at their own expense, a lying-in hospital and inaugurated full courses of lectures for the students. In 1815 James Hamilton (1767-1839) tried to persuade the Town Council and the University that training in midwifery should be compulsory for medical students. Gregory, the Professor of Medicine, and others in the Senate, fought this suggestion bitterly as they considered that the diseases of women and children were in the province of those who taught the practice of medicine. Not until 1824 did Hamilton win over the

8

Council. In 1830 the Senate was overruled and midwifery accepted as an essential part of the curriculum. James Hamilton, by establishing his subject in this way, brought the practice of obstetrics out of the darkness of superstition and out of the hands of the unqualified midwife. He resigned the Chair in 1839 and when James Simpson succeeded he was assured of a status equal to that of his colleagues in surgery and medicine.[5]

It has been suggested that the Edinburgh school was at its highest peak in the second half of the eighteenth century and that its status declined after 1800, never to be quite restored to its former glory. This is scarcely true because talent abounded in all branches of medicine from that date onwards and the influence of the school had spread far beyond Scotland. Admittedly the numbers fell from 1830 onwards and there were many attacks, often extremely virulent, on the quality of the teaching. The fall in numbers was in part due to the increasing size of the London schools, to the establishment of new schools in the provinces and to the greatly enhanced reputation of the Dublin school, which eventually rivalled Edinburgh in its attraction for English and foreign students. The rivals were in fact attaining the same standards, rather than the Edinburgh school declining in its standards.

There were many reasons for seeking a medical education in Edinburgh. It was not only that the school had absorbed the best of the continental teaching systems, that it abounded in men of great talent, but it was also that in England the modes of qualification were confused and usually more expensive. The qualifying degree in Edinburgh was an M.D. which carried a greater status than the M.R.C.S. of the London College or the License of the Apothecaries. Doctorates in medicine from the two ancient foundations of Oxford and Cambridge were obtained largely on theoretical knowledge and were not open to those who did not profess the established Church of England. Edinburgh, in contrast, opened her doors to all and offered a much wider practical and theoretical instruction. From 1750 onwards increasing numbers of Edinburgh graduates permeated all branches of the profession in all parts of the world. The London schools, inbred although they often tended to be, received much new

9

blood from Edinburgh. Charles Bell (1774-1842) and Henry Halford (1766-1844) of the Middlesex, Richard Bright (1789-1858) and Thomas Addison (1793-1860) of Guy's, Robert Liston (1794-1847) of U.C.H., William Fergusson (1808-1877) of Kings, were a few of the London men who qualified or studied in Edinburgh. The provincial schools, mostly founded in the nineteenth century, were infiltrated by Edinburgh graduates. To Liverpool came Joseph Brandreth (1746-1815), John Rutter (1762-1838) and James Carson (1772-1843). To Manchester came Charles White (1728-1813). Abraham Colles (1773-1843), Philip Crampton (1777-1858), Dominic Corrigan (1802-1880), Robert Graves (1787-1853) and William Stokes (1804-1878), all men of exceptional ability, raised the Dublin school to eminence. Many of the great American schools were modelled on Edinburgh and developed by her graduates, such as Benjamin Rush of Philadelphia.

In the nineteenth century the number of doctors in the army and navy was extremely high. Many were Scottish or Irish graduates and from Edinburgh the navy acquired men such as Gilbert Blane (1749-1834), Thomas Trotter (1760-1832), William Burnett (1779-1861) and John Richardson (1787-1865), all of great distinction. To the army went Robert Jackson (1750-1827) and James McGrigor (1771-1851) to name only two well-known army surgeons. John Lizars was in the navy and Robert Knox in the army for several years before settling in Edinburgh.

The list is endless and with many such names are associated major discoveries and advances in medicine and surgery. It was inevitable that all these men would show their loyalty to their parent university by ensuring that a promising student would go to Edinburgh for some phase of his medical education. Thus William Sharpey (1802-1888), Professor of Physiology in University College Hospital, advised the young Joseph Lister to complete his surgical training in Edinburgh under Syme. Family traditions developed by which succeeding generations returned for an Edinburgh degree. The impetus given to the Edinburgh school by the first Monro was thus perpetuated.

A medical school must be associated with a suitable hospital so that clinical instruction can be adequately pursued. In

1738 the foundation stone of the Royal Infirmary was laid. It was equipped to accommodate 228 patients and there was a large theatre in which as many as 200 students could view operations. The building of the hospital, completed in 1748, was a notable example of voluntary effort not only in terms of subscriptions from rich and poor, but also in the readiness and enthusiasm with which local merchants and craftsmen supplied free material and labour. In 1829 the building of the old High School was acquired as an extension and became the surgical hospital. This was to be the scene of much of the work of James Syme and Joseph Lister. The Infirmary transferred to its present site after 1870.[6]

In 1748 organised clinical lectures were first given in the Infirmary, although the provision of a theatre seems to suggest that the needs of teaching were considered when the hospital was first planned. Numerous private or semi-private hospitals sprang up and survived for varying periods, as for example, the lying-in hospital founded by the Hamiltons. Special hospitals were unusual at this time except for the Royal Edinburgh Asylum for the Insane founded in 1809 by the efforts of Professor Andrew Duncan.

Most clinical instruction from about 1750 to 1850, in all branches of medicine, was conducted in the Royal Infirmary. Some teachers, such as Syme, established small hospitals as private ventures and taught students in these during the intervals when they had no beds in the Infirmary.

Nursing was primitive until after 1860 when the influence of Florence Nightingale permeated to all hospitals. Before this date nurses were little more than domestics or orderlies, recruited from the lowest social scale and usually dirty, disorderly and often drunken. Occasionally a superior woman emerged, like the domineering but highly capable Mrs Porter who served both Syme and Lister. She earned immortality in the lines of the poet Henley:[7]

> Patients and students hold her very dear,
> The doctors love her, tease her, use her skill.
> They say the Chief himself is half afraid of her.

But Mrs Porter was the exception and the care of very ill patients often devolved on the students appointed to the

11

wards. They not only clerked meticulously on each case, but worked in shifts to nurse the very ill, particularly at night when there was no one else available. Dresserships accordingly offered an intensive and valuable training. An attachment to one of the more famous clinicians was sought avidly and often was a passport to later advancement.

The medical community was close-knit and revolved around the Infirmary, the Medical School, the two Royal Colleges and the medical societies. Of the latter the Royal Medical Society was of great importance. Evolving from a private debating club of students founded in 1737 and receiving a Royal Charter in 1779 this was the platform not only for the student but for the young graduate. The honour of election to the position of President was eagerly pursued and the influence and quality of the society was far beyond that of any other such student organisation. There were numerous other societies such as the Medico-Chirurgical founded in 1821; these provided ample means of communication in all branches of medicine, gave opportunities for good fellowship and even riotous pleasure and to belong to them gave prestige. Many of the doctors had wider interests and were members of the Philosophical Society or the Royal Society of the city. Simpson carried on this tradition when he became an active and prominent member, and later vice-president, of the Society of Antiquaries of Scotland.

There were local journals which began with the short-lived *Edinburgh Medical Essays* in 1731 and the *Medical and Philosophical Commentaries* in 1773. In 1805 the first number of the *Edinburgh Medical and Surgical Journal* was published to survive until 1953. These journals were, in general, of high standard and were contributed to not only by the local profession but by distinguished writers from other schools. Although critical they were comparatively free from the exploitation of slander and jealousy which characterised the contemporary London medical periodicals. The *Edinburgh Monthly Journal of Medical Science* was not guiltless in this respect for it was at times used to fan the quarrels of the day, or to print the propaganda of its 'conductors' or editorial board.

The progress and work of the Edinburgh school received due notice in the London journals although, particularly with the *Lancet* and the *Medical Times,* contributions from Edinburgh men were accepted more in relation to the personal likes and dislikes of the editors than to the quality of the productions. In 1828 in the first number of the *London Gazette* the editor wrote of a current view that 'no weekly paper will succeed which is not seasoned with personal abuse—we hope not to do so'. In fact the *London Gazette* proved as abusive as any periodical, in particular in its attacks on the *Lancet.* These editorial wars did not enhance the quality of medical literature and reflected the unseemly behaviour of the doctors of the time.

The output of monographs and larger works on all medical subjects was enormous. This may have been in part an indication of the gradual discard of the classical text books, sometimes in Latin, books which were the bibles of medical thought and practice, often relatively unchanged over the years. Edinburgh contributed more than a proportionate share to this output, aided by the great activity of Edinburgh publishers and printers. Many Edinburgh text books became popular and influential far beyond Scotland. In particular, in the first half of the nineteenth century, the most successful treatises on surgery emanated from Edinburgh, from the pens of those such as the Bells, Syme and Miller.

It is interesting to seek a comparison between early Edinburgh and London schools. In London the heterogeneous individual schools based on the ancient hospitals had little in common but rivalry. There was no parent university to co-ordinate medical education. The physicians and surgeons of London might be brilliant, but their talents were exerted very often towards the acquisition of wealth and social elevation by the cultivation of a fashionable practice. Their scientific contributions were often marred by personal jealousies and by offensive criticism in the current journals. The staffing of the hospitals was by nepotism and jobbing. Much of Wakley's fiery and vituperative writings in the *Lancet* were against these practices. The quality of training in the London schools varied greatly and the system of teaching was inferior to that in Edinburgh. The mushroom-like growth of the private schools in London testified to the inadequacy of the instruction in the old hospitals.

Astley Cooper, who was to become one of the greatest of the London surgeons, visited Edinburgh in 1787, admitted the superiority of teaching methods there and testified that in Edinburgh he learnt the diagnostic methods and skills which stood him in good stead throughout his career. He did think, however, that the London surgeons were better operators! An anonymous writer in the *Lancet* of 1837 visited the North and was unstinting in his admiration of the Royal Infirmary as a teaching hospital and compared London methods of instruction unfavourably.[8]

A survey of the medical scene in which Simpson and Syme were to play such great parts would be incomplete without some comment on the more general attitudes and behaviour of the doctors of the era. Unfortunately the *odium theologicum* had its counterpart, and its equal, in the *odium medicum*. Medical polemics are as old as medicine itself and may have reached a peak with the bitter controversies of the followers of Galen and those of Arabian medicine. In the Middle Ages the committal of a rival's medical works to the flames paralleled the public burning of heretical religious writings. Even martyrdom was occasionally the reward of the physician who advanced a new idea which upset established medical dogma. In later days the quarrels over a new development such as vaccination reached bitter heights. The work of Jenner was castigated by men like Rowley who manufactured quite incredible evidence against vaccination by relating tales of the acquisition of bovine characteristics in those who had been vaccinated, the woman who could no longer speak but mooed like a cow, the boy who developed an excrescence on his face like a bull's horn. In a profession which has always, and perhaps wisely, favoured cautious conservatism, there was a place for intense argument before established dogma was overthrown. Unfortunately most of these arguments were debased by the way in which the protagonists sank to personal abuse. Soon the original subject of the argument was forgotten and petty and trivial matters were pursued. In Edinburgh medical circles this quarrelsome atmosphere was present to an almost excessive degree. Perhaps it was a reflection of the times and was as marked in other professions, but it did not enhance the reputation of the doctors with their fellow citizens. It was not without justification that the counsel for the defence opening the case of Syme *v.* Lizars in 1840 used the following words. 'Few medical men can bear to know the soundness of their opinions has been questioned: they regard any such attempt as a signal of deadly personal hatred and view it in the same light as if their moral character had been questioned.' In 1858 Laycock, the newly appointed Professor of Medicine in Edinburgh, pleaded 'Are our professional brethren of Edinburgh always to live in an atmosphere of intrigue and hatred towards each other?' Simpson himself, then an ill and tired man, wrote to a friend in 1867: [9]

> ... we should be a profession of gentlemen and disputes should be settled as among gentlemen ... as I grow older I begin to think the kinder one is to some classes of minds the more bitter is their ingratitude. ...

In Edinburgh this regrettable disease was inherited in an acute form from the late eighteenth century. Gregory, the Professor of Physic, had published no less than eight large volumes of attacks on individuals and corporations. In 1792 there appeared an anonymous pamphlet entitled 'Guide to gentlemen studying medicine at the University of Edinburgh'. This was highly critical of all the professors except that of midwifery. Gregory, perhaps not surprisingly, accused Hamilton of writing the pamphlet and thrashed him with his walking stick. This cost Gregory £100 in damages. In the Senate Hamilton denied authorship of the pamphlet and Hope, the Professor of Chemistry, called him a liar. Hamilton sought £500 damages and was awarded one farthing. When Hope paid up he demanded a receipt. It was all very petty and the personal attacks extended even towards poor Mrs Hamilton who was publicly stated to be unsuitable as a member of a subscription ball, being the wife of an accoucheur. At a later date when Hamilton pressed for the establishment of midwifery on equal terms with surgery and medicine he was slandered, this time by Dr Duncan. Duncan went too far and was sued for £5,000; Hamilton received £50. Some people, not least the lawyers, found all this very profitable.

Such quarrels and litigations were so frequent that they were accepted as part of life and perhaps even enjoyed. They were fomented by public utterances in front of patients or colleagues, by letters in the lay and medical press often anonymous or under ill-disguised pseudonyms. Scathing pamphlets were exchanged and circulated. Most attacks were personal but the Infirmary, the Senate and the Colleges received a full share. In London the same kind of quarrels occurred, particularly because of the rivalries of the hospitals, but also because sides were taken so frequently by the editors of the journals. Things may have been rather worse in Edinburgh for the city was small enough for everyone to know the other's business; gossip spread like wildfire and a new cause erupted with surprising speed.

There was a more attractive side to the profession. From the previous century there had been bequeathed a tradition of conviviality and hospitality. Although not affluent in comparison with many of their London brethren the Edinburgh doctors lived well. Perhaps as a reaction to the austerity of life after the Reformation the city became in the eighteenth century a hive of social activity. There were dinners and balls, at which behaviour had to follow a meticulous protocol and private suppers and assemblies in taverns, where the wine flowed freely. Conversation was lively and embraced every topic. In all these gay occasions the doctors participated joining their colleagues from other faculties and mixing with the legal profession. The age did not lack characters. 'Lang' Sandy Wood, a cheerful surgeon of the day, visited his patients accompanied by a pet sheep and a raven. Professor Hamilton continued to visit his patients in a sedan chair up to 1830. John Bennet astonished the populace by driving his guests from dinner in a tavern in Leith to the theatre in a cortège of mourning coaches proceeding at an appropriately slow pace! Dr Graham, after establishing his quack 'Temple of Health' in London, returned to Edinburgh to lecture to the public on the preservation of health dressed in a white linen suit and black stockings. He was escorted by a retinue of servants in sumptuous livery, while Vestina, who subsequently became Lady Hamilton, posed on a pedestal to illustrate his talk! Only in Edinburgh could it happen that at the British Medical Association annual meeting in 1858 the tedium of the after dinner speeches was broken by three eminent professors singing glees.

What was the impact of this background on the young Simpson and the young Syme? Wordsworth had written in 1805:

> Bliss was it in that dawn to be alive
> But to be young was very heaven!

The words referred to the French Revolution but could well be applied to the period in general. But for Simpson and Syme there was another background. Over the city loomed the grey forbidding mass of the castle often obscured by the swirling mists of the North Sea and strangely divorced from the elegant streets and terraces of the New Town. To some the castle might represent the dour, uncompromising, proud and often belligerent people who had lived beneath it for hundreds of years. This was a people too with a sombre and serious strain, the inheritance of a struggle against extreme poverty and to some extent the sequel of an excessive reaction in Scotland to the Reformation. In many ways these national characteristics were antagonistic to the new age. Simpson and Syme responded in different ways to the two strong influences in their environment. On the one hand Simpson was sensitive to the new spirit. His character and temperament were such that he could enjoy living to the full and his ebullient spirit was such that he could rise to the heights of hope and happiness or sink to the depths of despair. A simple and happy childhood may have had much influence on the moulding of his character and it is tempting to speculate that the trace of French blood in his ancestry made him a little different from his more stolid fellow Scots. Syme on the other hand seemed deeply infused with the dominant characters of his race being cautious, conservative, reserved and at times unforgiving. But in their different manners both men had much to give and their careers were to reveal a curious contrast and to involve a violent clash of personalities which continued until they died in 1870.

CHAPTER 2

Early Life of Syme (1799-1828)

J OHN SYME, Writer to the Signet, lived in the New Town.
His family spent the autumn and winter at 56 Princes Street
and passed the summer at a country place in Kinross-shire.
Some of the houses of the New Town were laid out on the
north side of Princes Street but they did not have the style
of those built later in the squares and terraces on the ridges
between the castle and the sea. None of these early Princes
Street houses survives and the birthplace of James Syme can
be identified only as a site now occupied by a hotel. The street
was dramatically placed with the backdrop of the Castle Rock
and the fantastic silhouette of the Old Town lying to the
south. No building was at first permitted on the south side,
but this imaginative arrangement was rather spoilt for many
years because in between the Old and the New Town lay
the noisome, stagnant marsh of the Nor' Loch, the depository
of all the refuse of the ancient city. In time the Princes
Street proprietors were authorised by the City Corporation
to drain the loch, 'for the purpose of laying out the same, in
whole or in part, in a garden'. This difficult task was largely
accomplished by 1820 and the elegantly planted gardens
became the property of the tenants of Princes Street, whose
access was controlled by the possession of private keys. The
privilege was jealously guarded although an exception was
made in the case of Sir Walter Scott to whom the proprietors
granted a key so that he might enjoy the amenities. In 1826
the gardens were encroached upon by the creation of Playfair's
galleries built at the foot of the Mound, which linked the
old and the new city. The greater desecration, in the minds
of most, was the extension in 1846 of the Edinburgh and Glasgow railway from Haymarket, the original terminus, to the

east end of Princes Street. This and other influences soon converted the street from a residential to a commercial boulevard, while the private garden became a public park.[10]

When John Syme lived in Princes Street the area was fashionable and appropriate for one of the legal profession, of some wealth and of social position. He had married Barbara Spottiswood, also of good family, from Stirlingshire. The Symes had two sons, David, who followed his father's calling and James, who was born almost certainly at 56 Princes Street. In 1870, when Syme died, obituaries in two Edinburgh papers stated respectively that he was born in Fife or in Kinross-shire. That Edinburgh can claim the honour of his birthplace is confirmed by an entry in the Register of Births and Baptisms which reads: 'John Syme Esqr. W.S and Mrs Barbara Spottiswood his spouse St Andrews Church Parish a Son Born 7th Novem. 1799 names James. Witnesses the Revd Mr Henry Lister and Mr John Lister Writer Edinburgh'.[11]

There is nothing to suggest that John Syme achieved distinction in his chosen profession. He had private means which permitted him to give only intermittent attention to his legal work and to spend long periods in the country. He is credited as a man of 'much acuteness and sagacity; he was obstinate to a degree, the principle attribute of his character may be said to have been perseverance. . . .' Such attributes were undoubtedly transmitted to his son James but were unfortunately marred in the father by a tendency to indulge in reckless speculation. As was common at the time this was directed towards the purchase of land in the hope that values would increase with the discovery of minerals under the surface. John Syme's character was such that if he embarked on a venture he was unlikely to give it up even though failure was clear to all others. As a result his private fortune diminished and by 1808 he had given up his legal work in Edinburgh and removed to Kinross-shire. He continued his speculations with disastrous results and in 1813 sold his estate at Lochore in Fife and his family home at Cartmore in Kinross. He rented a rambling house at Pitreavie near Dunfermline and this was the family home until he died in 1821.

Despite all these troubles the Symes probably lived in fair

comfort during the boyhood of James and certainly there were adequate resources to provide for his education. If the father's speculations had any direct effect this was perhaps to impress on the son's mind the need for caution and care in money matters. In his life-time James Syme avoided any major financial difficulties while in contrast Simpson, brought up in poverty, became the reckless speculator.

The family lodged intermittently in Edinburgh during the period of James' school education. He attended initially a small private school in George Street and in October, 1805, entered the High School of Edinburgh. The school had been founded in the sixteenth century and to it went the sons of the Edinburgh middle and upper classes. The teaching was adequate although the classes were extremely large; James joined a group of 130 in his first year. He was too late to come under an exceptional rector, Alexander Adam, who had in his charge boys such as Francis Jeffrey, Walter Scott, Francis Horner and Henry Brougham, all of whom were to make their mark. There was brutality from some of the masters and the language and behaviour of many of the pupils were coarse. James seems to have been a silent, shy boy with few friends. His shyness may have been associated with an impediment in his speech. Rather unkindly Mr Pillans, the rector of the school, assumed that his defective utterance was adopted to avoid lessons; others were more sympathetic and helped him to overcome the disability. His work was consistent rather than brilliant and his favourite subject was chemistry. When the Syme family was in the country James lived in lodgings under the care of a private tutor Mr Simpson, later the Rev. Simpson. Just how much of James' education came from the school and how much from his tutor is difficult to decide. Perhaps the tutor was concerned mainly with his ward's religious and moral upbringing. Although shy, James was not unpopular at school and even amongst his rougher companions he acquired a reputation for his skill in performing chemical experiments. He left the school with fair credit and Paterson, his biographer, writes that on the final day James gathered up his school books and announced, 'Away with these toys: I am now done with them: the more serious business of life is before me, and to it I mean to address myself.' To a Victorian biographer this was just the incident, apocryphal or otherwise, to record and to testify, in hindsight, that the remark was 'an augury of the future'. One hopes he never spoke quite so smugly, but the story at least hints at a rather heavy and serious young man.

At the age of 16, in November 1815, James Syme matriculated in the University and at this stage there was no strong suggestion that he would study medicine. As a schoolboy he had spent his holidays in the country and interested himself in nature study and botany. Such pursuits were common to many boys of the time when organised sports were unusual. His love for botany persisted as perhaps his only real relaxation throughout his life.

Syme studied Latin under Professor Christison, father of his schoolfellow Robert who also was to become a professor in the University. He took out classes also in botany, natural history, mathematics and philosophy. Botany and philosophy were his favourite subjects and he pursued independently his interest in chemistry. Eventually Syme joined the chemistry class under Professor Hope, a man of brilliance who discovered the element strontium, but even with him the practical study of chemistry was not well organised and no experiments were performed by the students. Before Syme entered the chemistry class in 1817 he established a chemical society with a dozen friends, including Robert Christison. They met in different attics or cellars in their homes or elsewhere. Each member took his turn to demonstrate experiments and there was a predilection for the more dramatic and explosive varieties. Not surprisingly the society was usually asked to move on for at least on one occasion the demonstrator saved himself by diving under the table while his audience fled by the door. These activities were not very scientific but were at least original and Christison later recorded that the practical experience was of great value to him in his subsequent career.

Syme's chemical studies were rather more intensive than is suggested by the activities of his society. He must have read deeply beyond the requirements of the chemistry class. In March 1818 he wrote to the editor of the *Annals of Philosophy*: [12]

I take the liberty of sending you an account of a valuable substance which may be obtained from coal tar.

If you think it worthy of being made public, you will oblige me by inserting it in your *Annals of Philosophy*.

He forwarded a brief account of how he had distilled coal tar and obtained two liquid products. He had redistilled the supernatant fluid and derived a pure form of naphtha which he found was a solvent of white rubber, superior to any existent solvent. Although he hinted at practical applications he did not describe in the article that he had used the process to waterproof silk and other materials. He had, however, astonished his friends by treating a silk cloak so that it afforded absolute protection against rain and that it could be 'employed as a pitcher by turning up its skirt'.

His short paper was published in August 1818 and some of his friends appreciated the importance of the discovery. Syme himself dismissed the opportunity for wealth rather loftily as he 'was then about to commence the study of a profession with which considerations of trade did not seem consistent'. Perhaps he regretted this decision later when in 1823 the Glasgow chemist Charles Macintosh (1766-1843) received the credit for inventing a somewhat similar waterproofing process, thus immortalising his name and making a fortune from the patent. Writing in later years Syme recalled 'For my own part I gained little credit and no profit by the discovery, except the confidence which results from successfully struggling with difficulty, and encouragement in endeavouring to accomplish other objects of utility'. Syme was hard-headed and it is a little surprising that he failed to exploit the discovery. As a student he may not have appreciated what he might have gained by patenting the process but in his maturity he must have realised what an opportunity he had missed. It must be granted that the discovery was a remarkable one to be made by a mere boy working alone with primitive apparatus. It was evidence of originality and the ability to undertake a specific and difficult scientific research.

When Syme joined the University chemistry class in 1817 he had by then decided on a medical career, for in the same session he began the study of anatomy. He may have been influenced by Robert Liston (1794-1847) who was a distant relative. Like many others Syme sought instruction in anatomy in the extramural school under Barclay, the university lectures from Monro *tertius* having fallen into disrepute. Robert Liston was at this time one of Barclay's most able demonstrators but in 1818 they quarrelled and parted company. Liston formed his own anatomical class and Syme went with him to act as his assistant and demonstrator. He was very young and quite inexperienced for the task of teaching and controlling a class of 60 students but Liston gave every encouragement and his assistant was soon well thought of as a student teacher.

He had to attend other classes and his anatomical work could not occupy all his time. It is probable that he studied under the professors of the time, medicine under Duncan, surgery under Russel and Thomson and midwifery under Hamilton. He may well have attended some of the classes of the better teachers in the extra-mural school.

Before he qualified Syme was appointed to the Edinburgh Fever Hospital. This was administered by the Royal Infirmary and had been established in the Queensberry House Barracks to provide accommodation for the large number of patients smitten in the repeated epidemics of typhus and other fevers. A superintendent, two physicians and two physician-clerks were appointed to the hospital. Syme and his boyhood friend Robert Christison held the latter posts. There was a considerable risk of catching the prevailing fevers and many students and doctors working in this hospital succumbed. Syme suffered a serious illness from some unknown fever at this time but survived. When he recovered he obtained a resident clerkship in the Royal Infirmary under William Newbigging (1769-1852). Newbigging was President of the College of Surgeons in 1814; he received a knighthood in 1838 but has no particular place in surgical history. This was Syme's first real introduction to practical surgery and he was quick to observe the defects of much of the contemporary treatment. In particular he soon became aware of the excessive use of venesection in surgical cases including, ironically, those in whom there had been severe blood loss. The young house-surgeon dared to withhold venesection in the case of a debilitated boy with a compound fracture and instead he ordered porter and steak. This sensible prescription was quickly cancelled by an irate and orthodox chief. The vene-section controversy was to go on for many years and Syme was certainly one of the first to fight against its wholesale and illogical employment.

In April 1821 he passed the examination for the M.R.C.S. of London. It was a little unusual for an Edinburgh man to take this degree but one object may have been to secure recognition in London of any classes in anatomy or surgery which he might conduct. Perhaps too he looked forward to a day when, like so many of his countrymen, he would cross the Border and establish himself in London. That he did acquire the English diploma at this early stage may well have influenced the College to elect him as a Fellow in 1843 when some 300 were created without examination. Of these Fellows Syme was one of three surgeons practising in Edinburgh.

On completing his term of office as a resident in the Infirmary, Syme returned to the teaching of anatomy and collaborated with Liston for whom he often deputised. In the summer of 1822 he paid a visit to Paris. There the opportunities for anatomical dissection were better than in London and Edinburgh. Both these schools were woefully short of anatomical subjects and this deficiency was revealed by the exposure of a sinister traffic in corpses, culminating in the trial of the murderers Burke and Hare in 1828. Long before this crisis the anatomy schools had to acquire their material by dubious methods. Liston was a tough character possessed of great physical strength and there are many accounts which substantiate that he played an active part in body-snatching expeditions. There is no suggestion that Syme ever accompanied Liston on such adventures to the churchyards around Edinburgh.

Syme joined William Sharpey (1802-1880) an Edinburgh graduate, in Paris and a friendship started which continued for life. They attended the Paris hospitals and studied under Lisfranc and Dupuytren. Syme spent a lot of time doing comparative anatomy and prepared dissections of the skeletons of small animals so ably that the Paris naturalists thought he had a secret process of denuding the bones. At this stage he may have believed that his future lay in the teaching of anatomy,

24

especially as Liston was now concentrating more and more on surgical practice.

The months were spent in Paris perfecting anatomical knowledge but also learning much from the French surgeons whose technique was greatly in advance of others. When Syme returned to Edinburgh he continued to teach anatomy but also entered surgical practice. In 1823 he presented himself for the Fellowship of the Royal College of Surgeons and his dissertation on *Necrosis* was accepted. It was dedicated to Liston.

It soon became apparent that although he was prepared, like others, to go on devoting a lot of time to the teaching of anatomy, his sights were set on establishing himself as a surgeon. He could achieve this, as many had done before, by establishing a reputation in private practice, operating on patients in their homes or in hired premises which scarcely merited the title of private hospital. As a Fellow of the College he might hope, in due course, for a turn of office as surgeon to the Infirmary. To advertise himself he could lecture in surgery as well as anatomy, publish papers in the journals and take part in the activities of the medical societies.

He had scarcely embarked on his surgical career when he burst into the headlines with the news of an operation of considerable magnitude and importance. The *Edinburgh Medical and Surgical Journal* reported briefly in October 1823 that for the first time in Scotland a successful amputation at the hip joint had been performed. A full report by Syme appeared in the next number in January, 1824. The patient was William Fraser, aged 19, who had a painful, progressive disease of his femur. From the description this is likely to have been a chronic osteomyelitis or a tuberculous condition. Syme persuaded the boy and his parents that the leg should be amputated at the level of the hip joint, an operation seldom performed previously and very rarely attended by survival. Where he did the operation is unknown but he had the support of Dr Abercrombie at the consultation and of Liston at the operation. Syme's coolness and detailed anatomical knowledge were such that he fashioned the skin-flaps, severed the muscles and ligaments and removed the limb in less than a minute. Liston controlled the femoral artery by pressure in the groin, while Syme hastily changed his original plan of action because of difficulty in positioning the patient. The operation was not completed with the removal of the limb. It was not difficult to secure the main femoral vessel but the residual bleeding was torrential: [13]

> It seemed at first sight as if the vessels which supplied so many large and crossing jets of arterial blood could never all be closed. It may be imagined that we did not spend much time admiring this alarming spectacle; a single instant was sufficient to convince us that the patient's safety required all our expedition, and in the course of a few minutes haemorrhage was eventually restrained by the application of ten or twelve ligatures.

There was, of course, no anaesthetic and there is no comment on the reaction of the patient! Perhaps, mercifully, he fainted. The wound healed in a month and the operation was regarded as a success. Syme felt no hesitation 'in recommending it to the serious attention of operating surgeons . . . although it be the greatest and bloodiest in surgery: for I am sure that there is sometimes no other mode of prolonging existence.' With pride he wrote to Dr Sharpey on September 6th: [14]

> You will not be sorry to learn that one of your most particular friends has performed a great and grand operation which has thrown the good town . . . into commotion, and made him quite a notorious character.
>
> Little did I think, when slicing to pieces old Lisfranc's subjects, that I should have to perform amputation at the hip joint, far less that I should do it in Edinburgh on the 1st of September 1823: and if possible still less that I should do so with success. Yet all this has happened. . . .
>
> Nothing could have happened more fortunately than the affair occurring just now. I do hope he may recover; but, whatever way the matter ends, it must be favourable to me. . . .
>
> You will excuse me for being thus particular; for I know that, next to a man's own actions, those of his friends interest him most.

Unfortunately the patient died 10 weeks after the operation. But he survived long enough for Syme to derive justifiable credit and fame, as he hoped he would. In Edinburgh his name was made and the whole performance was to be typical of his future confidence, boldness and technical skill. He had modelled the procedure on what he had learnt from the Paris surgeons but did not hesitate, at a moment's notice, to alter established technique when he found complicating factors. The news reached London but the *Lancet* was not very flattering and compared the operation unfavourably with a recent similar success by Astley Cooper. There may have been some jealousy here and the comments were the beginning of a great deal of adverse criticism which was to flow from the *Lancet* against almost all that Syme attempted over the coming years.

The following summer, in 1824, Syme travelled to Germany for further post-graduate study and planned to spend four or five months. From a letter to Sharpey it appears that he was accompanied by a friend Dr Scott, with whom, in his methodical way, he studied German in preparation for the trip. There is no record of the visit nor is it clear under whom he studied in Germany.[15]

Meanwhile in 1823 Liston had given up active participation in his anatomy class and handed over his duties to Syme almost entirely. At first all went well and Syme retained a large and profitable class with Liston holding only a controlling interest. Just when everything seemed encouraging there was a quarrel. The origin of this is uncertain but it is very likely that Liston was becoming jealous of the success of his protégé not only as a teacher but also, and more so, of his rising reputation as a surgeon. There was not room for many successful consultants in the relatively small city and it was rumoured that there were misunderstandings over private patients. Further it seems likely that Syme disapproved of Liston's close collaboration with the body-snatchers, necessary although this might be to keep the dissecting room going. The partnership was broken and so was a friendship, only to be restored many years later when Liston was settled in London. It was a worrying period for Syme, for on the death of his father in 1821 the family estate had melted away in meeting heavy debts. Syme could not yet depend on his surgical practice to provide an adequate income and so he became attached to Dr Mackintosh in the newly founded

Brown Square extra-mural school of medicine. Syme delivered the lectures in anatomy and surgery and the school flourished initially. By January 1825 he reported to Sharpey that his own class was thriving; and a large class meant an assured source of income. He was becoming increasingly interested in the teaching of surgery whereas the teaching of anatomy brought him great problems in the supply of subjects for the dissecting room. Legislation against the illicit practices of the body-snatchers had been tightened but the Government of the day had offered no satisfactory alternative means of supply. Believing that it was easier to organise these matters in Ireland, Syme visited Dublin in 1826. In fact the situation in Ireland was even worse than in Edinburgh, as is related by John Crosse a Norwich surgeon who studied in Dublin at this time. The visit had the effect of hardening his intention to give up the teaching of anatomy and to take up surgery alone. He was particularly impressed by the work of the Dublin surgeon Cusack but admired all the surgical practice and teaching in this rising school.[16]

When he returned there was a rather trivial quarrel with his colleagues in Brown Square and as a result he severed his connection with this school. To the alarm of his friends and family he proposed to practise and teach surgery on his own despite the competition of well established men such as Liston, Lizars and Fergusson in the extra-mural schools and Thomson and Russel in the University. It was a bold decision but Syme was a determined character and when he had an objective he pursued it vigorously and relentlessly. He was hampered by the lack of a hospital appointment. Although a vacancy occurred in the Infirmary about this time the Managers would not appoint him, allegedly because they feared there would be public bickering with Liston.

Undaunted, Syme decided to establish a hospital of his own and nothing he achieved illustrates more clearly his energy and determination. At the age of 30 he was issuing a challenge to his seniors and to some the project appeared foolish. His own financial resources at the time were negligible but he sought to make the scheme viable by gaining the support of the public and by charging fees to pupils attached to the hospital. He selected Minto House near the University, on the site now occupied by Chambers Street. This was a large square building occupied by the Elliots of Minto until they, like other noble families, deserted the old city. He calculated that having obtained a long lease on easy terms he needed £300 to equip the building as a surgical hospital and £700 for its annual support. Two house surgeons were to pay £100 a year for the privilege of working with him and he hoped for student fees to the amount of £250 each year. The rest of the money had to come from private subscriptions or from his own pocket. It was encouraging that the University agreed to recognise his course of lectures in surgery and that the London College also accepted his teaching. A distinguished and influential body, headed by some titled gentlemen, was elected as a board of directors and soon £100 was raised in subscriptions. The appeal came to Liston's notice but he wrote in the book 'Don't support quackery and humbug'. Syme reacted immediately by raising an action for damages and litigation was avoided only when Liston wrote a humble letter of apology. Otherwise all went well and in May 1829 the hospital was staffed and equipped and open to poor patients who were treated free. The hospital flourished and established Syme without question as a rising surgeon in the city and more than compensated for his failure to get on the staff of the Infirmary.

From when Syme published his case of amputation at the hip joint, to 1829, a flow of papers came from his pen, most of which appeared in the Edinburgh journals. The most significant were his studies on wounds and inflammation, his first cases of excision of joints for tuberculosis and a remarkable report of the removal of a huge tumour of the lower jaw.

To assess the importance of these early contributions it is necessary to review briefly the state of surgery at the time. The field was narrow and attitudes were conservative. The treatment of acute inflammation was based on indeterminate theories, although there were already strong hints of the contagious nature of some diseases. Wounds and fractures formed a large proportion of the conditions for which patients were admitted to hospital and a compound fracture often resulted in the loss of a limb if not of a life. Amputations were done with great dexterity and speed but with a very high mortality rate. The management of fistulae and of bladder stones were specialised arts and the subject of much argument. Aneurysms were common and in their treatment heroic ligations of major vessels were done with meagre success. Large external tumours were attacked boldly but often with disaster from bleeding or sepsis. The abdominal cavity was rarely explored although in 1826 John Lizars, to the detriment of his reputation, attempted the removal of ovarian cysts on four occasions with at least one success. Various operations were attempted for hernia, usually for the acute case, but in general ill-founded theories, such as those which induced a fear of exposing the abdominal cavity to air, restricted these attempts. Obstruction of the bowel and peritonitis were usually managed by the physicians, who employed in particular a wide variety of enemata, ranging from tobacco-smoke to mercury, usually with disastrous results.

Up to about 1830 most of Syme's work represented extensions of existing techniques but his advocacy of joint excision rather than amputation for tuberculosis conditions was a notable advance which he was to develop further. Like many other surgeons he was disposed to attach too much importance to being the first to do a particular operation and did not appreciate that it was more important to take a new technique, to collect a series of cases and to follow this up to establish a principle. Even today the importance of 'firsts' can be greatly exaggerated: if arguments over priorities are vehement and petty then true advances are obscured.

Not many surgeons in this period were 'pure' surgeons, in fact in the coming years Syme was at great pains to impress on everyone that he was the only 'pure' in Scotland. Most of his colleagues practised some medicine and even midwifery. Most remained subservient to the physicians who, although they rarely operated themselves, expected to dictate to the surgeons as to when they should operate. The social status of the surgeon had, however, risen considerably from the time when he was so inferior to the physician that he used the servants' entrance of the great houses while the physician was received with due ceremony at the front door. In London it was now possible for the surgeon to rise to the heights of the social scale and in the process he often made a considerable fortune. The Edinburgh surgeons did not usually have such profitable practices.

Syme's assistant Peddie has left us a caricature drawn about 1830 and also a verbal picture: [17]

He was of short stature and slim, although in his later days stout in figure, his dress most unbecoming but that of the period—namely a black, long-tailed coat with stiff large collar, dark gray or black trousers, and a black and white checked neckcloth. His head was large and finely shaped, nose longish, eyes dark gray, large and penetrating, upper lip full and round, mouth firm—the least pleasant of his features, chin retreating, neck short and hands and feet beautifully formed and strong. His utterance was at times slightly stuttering, and his voice somewhat muffled, but his delivery was so serious and emphatic, his style so clear, concise and vigorous . . . that he was invariably listened to with close attention and interest. . . .

He never unnecessarily wasted a word, a drop of ink or of blood. . . .

By some he was considered short in temper—nay he has been spoken of as irritable, quarrelsome and cold-hearted, but those who said this could not have known him intimately . . . those who knew him best esteemed him well . . . ever activated by kind and humane feelings, deeply felt, though not effusively expressed.

The *Medical Times* printed a series of *Pencillings of Eminent Medical Men* and in 1844 it was Syme's turn to be portrayed. The description is not flattering, but allowing for the inaccurate, satiric and often cruel style of these sketches it must point to some truth concerning the impact of Syme on the superficial observer: [18]

Professor Syme overflows with benevolence, just as a hot frying pan spits back the cook's gift of water . . . He is a little man: of pale, sallow saturnine aspect: short neck: large heavy hanging lips and a mouth whose size suggests visions of oxen roasted whole. We mistake him or he could swallow every appointment in the University's gift . . . Edinburgh's shrewdness has well named him the serpent. . . . Were we Aberdeen or Palmerston we would secure his diplomatic aid at any price he fixed in it. National diplomacy will never be at its acme till it enlist the Edinburgh Professor of Clinical Surgery.

Of his letters in this early period few survive with the

exception of those to Sharpey. It is possible to read between the lines and to presume that Syme put all aside in his ambition to become a leader in surgery. He worked hard and it seems likely he had little time for jollity, that he was solemn and humourless and that, except to a limited circle of intimates, he was rather unapproachable.

Confident in his professional advancement Syme became married in 1829 to Miss Willis, the daughter of a Leith merchant and sister of an old school-fellow. Little is known of her but Paterson describes her as 'amiable, intelligent, accomplished and judicious and devoted to her domestic duties'. Two daughters survived from this marriage, the elder, born in 1835, was Agnes who married Joseph Lister in 1856. The first Mrs Syme died in 1840 and Syme re-married the following year. In 1826 Syme lived in 6 Forth Street, in 1828 he moved to 75 George Street, in 1830 to 2 Forres Street and in 1836 to 9 Charlotte Square.

James Simpson was born eleven years after Syme and was a student when Syme was well established as an extra-mural teacher in anatomy and surgery. Simpson studied these subjects under the University professors and attended the extra-mural classes of Lizars and Liston. It is unlikely that their paths crossed before 1830 but Simpson would be very much aware of Syme's rapid rise to fame.

CHAPTER 3

Early Life of Simpson (1811-1838)

J AMES SIMPSON was born on June 7th, 1811 in the town of Bathgate. Dr Dawson the local practitioner recorded in his day book 'Lab. nat. easy, rapid. 8th child. Son natus 8 o'clock. Uti veniebam natus. Paid 10s. 6d.' (In modern obstetric usage 'born before arrival'.) Some of his critics in the future were to affirm that he 'was always in a hurry'. An entry from the Register of Births and Baptisms for the Parish of Bathgate reads '1811 June 7th David Simpson and his spouse Mary Jarvey had a child born. Baptd. the 30th June James Simpson'. This confirms that he added the name Young soon after qualification as a doctor, an explanation is that because of his youthful appearance he was known to his friends simply as 'Young Simpson'.[19]

His grandfather, Alexander Simpson, was a farmer and farrier in the district and had married Isabella Grindlay whose great niece, Jessie Grindlay, became the wife of James Simpson. In 1810 his father, David Simpson, had settled in Bathgate as a baker and had married Mary Jarvey the daughter of a local farmer.

James Simpson's paternal forbears were men of strong character, energetic and able in their business of farming. The grandfather, Alexander Simpson, had particular skill in treating animal diseases but if his orthodox methods did not succeed he was ready to ascribe this to witchcraft and to fall back on expedients based on country superstitions. James Simpson, when he became an enthusiastic archaeologist, recalled family stories such as that of the burial alive of a healthy cow in order to arrest a cattle plague. On the maternal side the influences on James were more subtle. His mother's father

John Jarvey was descended from a Huguenot family which had settled in this part of Scotland some generations previously. He had married Mary Cleland whose family was of a higher social grade than his own. Through her James Simpson could trace a pedigree of some historical importance, although the evidence that he could claim descent from the Scottish hero William Wallace is somewhat tenuous.

David Simpson in his youth had been stirred to see the world and had walked to London with his brother in the hope of making a fortune. To the relief of the father, who feared his sons might be press-ganged, he soon returned to settle down in his native town as a baker. His affairs did not prosper until after the birth of James when Mrs Simpson took over the management of the bakery and established it profitably. It is clear that she was the dominant partner and although she died when James was nine she had a great influence upon him. James was the seventh son and there was a strong belief that as such he would bring good fortune to the family and that he would be a favoured child. Of the seven other children Mary was the eldest and when the mother died Mary brought up the younger members of the family. Of the six other sons one died in infancy while the elder brothers, particularly Alexander, were to prove great supports to James throughout all his life.

James was born in a small house in Main Street which lay on the coach route between Edinburgh and Glasgow. Although only 18 miles from the capital Bathgate was at the time an isolated village. There must, however, have been some excitement and news of the outside world when the daily coach lumbered through the cobbled streets of the town. The community numbered some 2,000 people and included a large number of handloom weavers who were men of exceptional intelligence and often self-educated to a remarkably high degree. They were quick-witted and took an active part in local and general political life. Religion loomed large in the life of the people but there were contrasting elements of immorality and drunkenness, all too usual in any small Scottish town. The neighbouring countryside was not yet marred by the development of mining and other industries. The family atmosphere was deeply religious and very happy.

34

James was inculcated by his mother with simple Christian beliefs from the Catechism and the Bible. The whole family united in their care of the youngest and all made sacrifices so that he would be well educated. In due course the traditional Scottish custom was followed by which the brightest member of the family was supported at university by his brothers who stayed on at home at their simple pursuits.[20]

Allowing for a degree of sentimentality in the accounts of the last century it does seem that James was a particularly attractive child: 'A rosy bairn wi' laughin' mou' and dimpled cheeks.' From an early age he took his share of helping in the bakery and delivering the bread but in general his path was smoothed so that he could get on with his studies, for which he at once showed great aptitude. He went to school at the age of four being taught at first by Mr Henderson who, having lost a limb, was known as 'Timmerlegs'. The village schoolmasters at the time were often such men who could not earn a living otherwise and whose academic attainments were often negligible. James was fortunate in that soon he continued his education with a Mr Taylor who was an exceptional schoolmaster. The small school in a short period produced three professors, James Simpson, John Reid, Professor of Anatomy at St Andrew's and the Rev. Dr John Fleming, Professor of Natural Science at New College.

The education at the village school must have been very basic and simple and James was soon head and shoulders above his classmates. His mother ensured that he absorbed all the knowledge he could from the scanty library of the household, with the Bible and other religious books predominating. Limited as his resources must have been he read widely and with great avidity. In the countryside there was opportunity for exploration and, like Syme, his interest was soon aroused in natural history. As a child James paid at least one visit to Edinburgh and a stirring of his future antiquarian interests was shown by a visit to Greyfriars' churchyard where he copied two inscriptions from the ancient tombstones.

Another boy from Bathgate, John Reid, had gone to the University two years before James left school. Simpson never forgot how impressed he and his friends were when John Reid returned home after his first term at college: [21]

35

We listened eagerly and wonderingly to what he told us of it, and particularly of the College and its Professors. But, like most others, I was on the whole less awestruck with this than with the strange metamorphosis which appeared to have mysteriously occurred in our former schoolmate, for the rough country schoolboy who had left us two short months before, had become suddenly changed into a sharpish college student, wearing an actual long-tailed coat, and sporting a small cane.

In 1825 James Simpson followed this local hero to university, at the tender age of 14, and he entered a world very different from that of the protective atmosphere of his simple home. His achievements in the village school meant little in a university class and the standards he had reached were such that he had a great many new subjects to master in his first year at college. He was entirely supported by his father and brothers and embarked on his student life in penurious circumstances. The rent of his lodgings was only three shillings a week but every penny had to be accounted for in his reckoning. While he did not starve his expenditure on the necessities of life was meagre and his only extravagance was in the purchase of books. In an entry in his diary may be seen the strange juxtaposition of 'Finnan Hadies 2d. Bones of the Leg £1. 1s. Subject £2. Spoon 6d. and Bread and Tart 1s. 8d. and "Early Rising" 9½d.' This indicates the simplicity of his diet and the heavy cost of anatomical study. The purchase of the pamphlet *Early Rising* reveals his early determination to plan his life with economy of time.[22]

He was not friendless and it was probably a great comfort to his family that he lodged with John Reid and an older student Macarthur who had taken up the study of medicine after being a teacher at Bathgate. That the family prodigy would enter the ministry was doubtless the hope of his father and brothers: it was to this end that many such simple Scottish families scraped the money together to support a promising boy at university. The contact with Reid and Macarthur decided things otherwise, for they allowed him to read their medical books and at an early stage took him to one of Robert Knox's stimulating lectures.

In his first session James studied Greek, Latin and mathematics, did well if not brilliantly in these subjects and was given a sound basic education before he concentrated on medicine. At the beginning of his second year he enrolled as a medical student and his financial situation was eased somewhat when he was awarded a bursary of £10 a year. He took out class tickets for anatomy under Monro and Lizars, for chemistry under Hope and Kemp, for botany under Graham and for natural philosophy under Lees. Like most students he depended on extra-mural instruction as well as on the official university courses. He studied surgery under Liston for whom he developed great admiration and for a period he acted as a dresser in Liston's wards in the Infirmary. He attended Hamilton's lectures in midwifery but confessed later that the subject did not interest him as a student and that he fell asleep at the lectures. All the time he was a student he took elaborate notes and the margins of these were sprinkled with question marks and 'why, why'. Right from the start he revealed an intensely critical mind and he was not afraid to challenge the established ideas of his teachers. His powers of observation were trained by his interest in natural history. In the holiday periods he studied geology, botany, zoology and meteorology in the Bathgate countryside and made meticulous notes of his observations.[23]

But for the companionship of his fellow students, most of whom were poor like himself, his amusements were few. That he was a dreamer is suggested by a few incursions into the writing of romantic poetry. Most of the time, however, he worked very hard and it was no surprise that he cleared his first major academic hurdle with comparative ease. He qualified L.R.C.S.Ed. in 1830, a month short of the age of 19. To advance himself further he was anxious to take the degree of M.D. but he was still too young to qualify for this.

The time had come for him to make a career and a living. His father died in the year that James qualified and his brothers John and Alexander took over the parental responsibilities. No doubt they felt that James should now capitalise on his expensive training and should settle in some post such as that of a country practitioner, which was after all to them a position of great dignity and respect. James may already have had higher ambitions but he was content to remain at home for the summer and to assist Dr Girdwood of Falkirk and the family doctor, Dawson, of Bathgate. His brother John wrote to Mr Grindlay of Liverpool, a relative of Mrs Simpson and a thriving merchant, asking him if he could place James as a ship's surgeon. But they were not going to allow the pride and joy of the family to run any risks, 'he is the youngest of us all, and a favourite, and we would be averse to his going in a ship designed for any unhealthy shore'. John Simpson must have known that ships' doctors on the West African run from Liverpool suffered a high mortality from cholera and the like and it was fortunate for humanity that Mr Grindlay did not immediately find a vacancy.

Meanwhile the family were prepared to go on helping James generously and he returned to Edinburgh in 1831. He worked for a while with Dr Gairdner in dispensary practice and Gairdner thought highly of his assistant's industry and ability. This period allowed Simpson time to prepare a thesis for the M.D. and he presented this, as was required at the time, in Latin, on the subject of 'Death from Inflammation'. About this year he applied for the post of surgeon at Inverkip, an insignificant Clydesdale village. He was rather hurt that he did not get the appointment and in later life often wondered, had he succeeded, whether or not he would have remained there for life in obscurity.

The fates had determined otherwise for his thesis was read by Thomson, the Professor of Pathology. He was impressed by the quality of the work of the young unknown and invited Simpson to become his assistant at £50 a year. The offer was timely for meanwhile Mr Grindlay of Liverpool had written with the chance of a ship's surgeoncy. Simpson however accepted Thomson's invitation with alacrity. By doing so it was assured that he would remain in Edinburgh in this active centre of medical thought and influence and that he would in time make his own great contributions there.

It was not long before Thomson suggested to his assistant that there was an opening in midwifery for an active young man. The hint was taken and very quickly Simpson immersed himself in the study of obstetrics and gynaecology. He attended again the lectures of the now ageing Hamilton and this time he listened, appreciating that Hamilton had a lot of sound wisdom and practical experience to impart. While

38

midwifery now became his most important activity he remained deeply interested in the wider fields of medicine and surgery. For a while he deputised for Thomson by giving the university lecture course in pathology. His concentration on this subject, then very much in its infancy as a separate branch of medicine, laid the foundation for much of importance in his later work.

The circumstances of his appointment are enlarged upon in a belated letter Simpson sent to Walter Grindlay in November 1832: [24]

> Long ere this time you will have been considering as somewhat extraordinary the absolute silence that has been preserved on the part of my brother John and myself, respecting the recommendation which you were so very good as send me for the surgeonship of the *Belsey* —Allow me to explain the reason, why no answer has hitherto been returned to you, to offer you at least all that we have at present in our power to offer— thanks for your kind remembrance of me.
>
> Your letter came of course, as it was addressed, to my brother John at Bathgate. He sent it to Edinburgh to me, as soon as possible after he received it, and as I happened to be very busily engaged for some days at that time my brother David who is in business as a Baker here went to Leith for me to advertise Mr. Petrie not to keep the situation you pointed out vacant on my account. . . .
>
> A word now as to the reason for my non-acceptance of the surgeonship of the *Belsey*. In taking my degree here last summer I had the good fortune to attract the notice of Dr John Thomson, a physician of the greatest eminence, who was then looking for a person to assist him in the composition of his lectures, which he is now for the first time delivering in this University as Professor of General Pathology. He offered me this situation wholly unsolicited and altogether unexpected on my part. I entered into it in July last and besides a moderate salary I enjoy every conceivable advantage for cultivating the most perfect knowledge of my professor and am used in most respects as one of his own family.

His preoccupation with his duties in the pathology department, however, began to worry him as he had now determined on a career as an obstetrician and competition was severe in the extra-mural school. He wrote in June 1838: [25]

It was decidedly an unfortunate step as I can now see that I took when I accepted the interim professorship of Pathology, I ought to have been lecturing for myself and by omitting to do so have allowed others to get started before me in that field.

Like Syme in his early career Simpson had to prove himself in his chosen subject. To do this he too began to teach in the extra-mural school, to participate in the meetings of the important societies, to acquire a private practice and to write for the journals. As far as his future was concerned his most important obstetrical paper in this period was on diseases of the placenta. Not only was this work highly regarded in Edinburgh, when he used it for his presidential address to the Royal Medical Society in 1835, but also it was translated into German and other languages and attracted considerable notice in the important schools in Europe.

In the short period of three years, while still a very young man, Simpson was becoming recognised as a new force. The science of obstetrics and gynaecology was not well established and, in general, these subjects were taught and practised by physicians and surgeons as sidelines. There was a confused situation, for the physician-accoucheur might well encounter conditions for which surgical operations were required but which he was not competent to perform. There was an inheritance of quackery and even superstition which influenced the management of childbirth and the unqualified, often disreputable, midwives still exerted considerable sway. It was only a matter of a hundred years since the presence of a male attendant at a birth was thought a monstrous thing. The obstetric forceps introduced by the Chamberlens in the early eighteenth century had remained a family secret for years. There was certainly scope for someone who could tidy up the confused teaching and practice of the day and a man of Simpson's intelligence and energy had a remarkable opportunity.

Between 1830 and 1836 there were lean years for Simpson but they paved the way to his ultimate triumphs. Without the help of his brothers he would not have survived except in some minor field of medicine. For a while he was able to live cheaply with his brother David who had a bakery business in Edinburgh. Alexander and John loaned him money to augment the small income he derived from teaching and from his few private patients.

A European tour was considered an essential part of the training of a rising specialist and once more the brothers came forward with their liberality. In 1835 with his friend Douglas MacLagan (1812-1900), later Professor of Medical Jurisprudence in Edinburgh, Simpson set out to visit some of the foreign medical centres. First of all there was a month in London. They attended at the important hospitals and the College of Surgeons and they did the sights such as the House of Commons, St Paul's Cathedral and the Surrey Zoological Gardens. It is typical of his curiosity and observation that in the Zoo he should notice that a lion had cataract in both eyes and that 'one monkey coughed severely—is it consumption?' In early May they crossed the Channel and travelled to Paris by coach. There they visited the main hospitals and met such notables as Baron Larrey, Lisfranc, Flourens and Dubois. They were greatly impressed by Dr Esquirol who had abolished coercive treatment in the asylum at Charenton. Not a moment was wasted but although they worked hard the sights of Paris were not neglected. He wrote to one of his cousins on the 23rd April giving his impressions of Paris, but his presbyterian blood was roused! [26]

The way in which Sunday is kept would astonish you. . . . Dr Moffatt and I went to the churches of St Rocques, Notre Dame and the Madeleine and saw the service—fearfully, fearfully catholic, with priests in the gayest possible gowns, long candles burning, bells ringing, women busily uttering prayers and men holding out everywhere brushes wet with holy water for you to touch.

In June the travellers visited Liège, Brussels, Antwerp and Ghent. Simpson made many contacts which were of value to him in the future and he took careful notes of all he saw. On the journey home there was a brief visit to Liverpool and an evening was spent with his relatives the Grindlays. He was immediately attracted to one of the daughters of the house and saw in her a resemblance to his much loved sister Mary. This was probably the first meeting with Jessie Grindlay who became his wife. [27]

The short foreign tour rounded off Simpson's experience

and education. By 1836 at the age of 25 he was now embarked on his life's work. His earnings might be insignificant but his reputation was rising fast both at home and abroad. In this year he was made a corresponding member of the Medical Society of Ghent, the first of many foreign honours. He was deeply involved in a variety of studies and from these he began to issue the flow of papers and pamphlets which persisted throughout his life. An appointment to the City Lying-in-Hospital in 1836 increased his clinical opportunities and, indirectly, his private practice. The ambition to reach the summit of his chosen profession must have developed strongly by this time. Both he and Syme must have realised that the ultimate aim must be the acquisition of a university chair in Edinburgh. Failing this, for both, there must always have been the alternative attraction of a move to the wider sphere of London.

Syme became Professor of Clinical Surgery in 1833 and Simpson Professor of Midwifery in 1840. The clash of their personalities did not develop until they were thrown together in the University Senate. Their personal contacts up to 1840 were probably limited to a casual acquaintance in the medical societies. Neither Simpson nor Syme found the path to their cherished ambition smooth and the events which lead to their appointments provide interesting sidelights on the academic rivalries, the jealousies and the pitfalls encountered by those who strove for advancement in the medical profession.

As a young man Simpson, although dedicated to his work, found time for the pleasures of life. He wrote to Jessie Grindlay in 1838: [28]

> Last winter was a strange blend of working and romping—of study and idleness—of pleasure and pathology—of lecturing and laughing—of investigating the phenomena of diseases and dinner parties—of agues and quadrilles—of insanity and co-quetry. I had everything in excess except sleep, and the paucity of it made room for the superfluity of everything else—good, bad and indifferent. If my head was clear enough to cast up the gains and losses . . . it would be in favour of the former.

Already his extreme restlessness was apparent and whether in his work or pleasure he was always intensely occupied. Perhaps he burnt the candle at both ends for he soon paid the penalty in attacks of depression and headaches. In 1836 he wrote to Jessie: [29]

> I have been on the sick list repeatedly since you left with headaches etc. etc.—and have been bled, leeched, salivated etc. etc.—I hate the intermeddlements of these folks yclept Doctors —they are really a great pest—and I a bad patient. I had six leeches behind the left ear and walked out after it. I have some ugly threatenings of an inflammation of the ear and was laid up with one for two months before when I first set off on the jaunt during which I first visited Liverpool for the recovery of my health. I had a plateful and a half of blood taken from me one night . . . I had my head leeched etc. on the Friday—and on coming home from my evening visits on the Sunday at 10 o'clock found a message ordering me off to Kirkcaldy. . . . Returned to Edinburgh about 6 on Tuesday evening went to bed for an hour with a swollen face and salivating mouth— rose at 8 and danced at a party of Mrs Walker's till my face was considerably better—that is till 3 a.m. on Wednesday morning when I came home and sat down to my lecture. . . .

The account is typical of his way of life yet he expressed regrets that he was not doing enough and he resented the loss of the very few hours he gave to sleep. His energy was exceptional and blessed with a powerful frame he could pack into the day and night far more than any ordinary mortal. He was a handsome young man despite a rather short, stout body and an exceptionally large head. It was his personality, however, which impressed people and when he died a vivid description was given of him when he presided at the Royal Medical Society about 1835: [30]

> The Chair was occupied by a young man whose appearance was striking and peculiar. As we entered the room . . . little was seen but a mass of tangled hair, partially concealing what appeared to be a head of very large size. He raised his head and his countenance at once impressed us. . . . A pale large, rather flattish face, massive, brent brows, from under which shone eyes now piercing as it were to your inmost soul, now melting into almost feminine tenderness, a coarseish nose, with dilated nostrils, a finely chiselled mouth, which seemed the most expressive feature of the face, and capable of being made at will the exponent of every passion and emotion. Who could describe that smile? . . .

There are other such descriptions which testify to Simpson's unique appearance and to his almost hypnotic influence on his fellow men and women.

CHAPTER 4

Professional Advancement (1828-1840)

SYME did not take long to make Minto House a centre which made the established surgeons of the Infirmary sit up and take notice. He appointed John Brown and Alexander Peddie as his house surgeons. John Brown (1810–1882) was the son of the minister of Biggar and like Syme he had been educated at the High School in Edinburgh. During his medical training he and his friend Peddie, were apprenticed to Syme. Brown delighted to recall how Syme with the apprenticeship fees was able to purchase his first carriage. Syme took his young assistant to try out this handsome gig with yellow wheels and with typical concentration on the task in hand he said, 'I make one rule, John; there will be no talk.' Brown became a fashionable and kindly physician and had a second profession as an author. His essays, rather heavily entitled *Horae Subsecivae*, and other writings, gained him a high reputation with the contemporary critics who rated him almost the equal of Charles Lamb. *Rab and his Friends* was a best seller and remains well known today. Written some 30 years after Brown worked with Syme at Minto House this simple human document presents vividly the atmosphere of the hospital, the characters of the protagonists from the surgeon to the heroic patient and the horrors of surgery before anaesthesia and antisepsis. It is related how a simple carrier brought his wife to consult Syme. The examination was brief but kindly and the verdict was given in a few words, that an operation must be done to try and cure her of a malignant tumour of the breast. Next day the students crowded the theatre and there was excitement at the prospect of a major operation. Ailie walked into the theatre and the unruly clamour was at once stilled by her dignity and courage. Her husband stayed with her during the ordeal. So did his faithful dog Rab, crouched in a corner with his ears cocked, suspicious of all that was happening. The operation was completed without a murmur from the patient but with an occasional growl from Rab. At the end Ailie was assisted from the table, she curtsied decorously to the surgeon and to the students and begged their pardon 'if she had behaved ill'. Tragically, but all too inevitably, she died in the delirium of septicaemia in a few days. The account is full of pathos and can be read and re-read in its entirety.[31]

John Brown remained a close friend and colleague of Syme and admired him greatly. He knew him better than most men and in later years they often went on holiday expeditions together. Brown gives a much more kindly and sympathetic picture of Syme than does any other of his contemporaries, except perhaps Syme's son-in-law Lister, and was one of the few who seems to have penetrated the external harshness and coldness of his character. Through Brown, Syme had some acquaintance with the literary figures of the time for Brown was an intimate of writers such as Thackeray and Ruskin. There were many letters from Ruskin to 'My Dearest Dr Brown'.[32]

Alexander Peddie, the second of the house surgeons at Minto House, although less famous than John Brown, became President of the Royal College of Physicians. He too remained a close friend and colleague of Syme and cared for him in his last illness.

The surgical work at Minto House was chronicled in great detail by Syme in a series of reports from 1829 to 1833. These quarterly accounts appeared in the *Edinburgh Journal* and most were annotated in the London journals. From them it is clear that Minto House attracted patients from all over Scotland and that Syme operated for all sorts of conditions to achieve results which probably were very much better than those of his rivals in the Infirmary. At first he recorded interesting or unusual cases but in time he devoted all or part of each report to the substance of a lecture on a specific problem. In this way he advertised his work and his teaching methodically.

Not surprisingly some regarded Syme as an upstart and

when Minto House was closed an anonymous correspondent to the *Edinburgh Journal* was scornful of the 'Minto House Yarns' and gratified that Syme could now 'turn his attention from the quantity to the quality of his cases'. Another critic, in the *Lancet*, accused Syme of habitual inaccuracy in his case reports, 'in future we shall know what credit to attach to "Reports by Professor Syme" '. 'Studens Scotus,' affirming that Syme 'had made a botch of an amputation' wrote scathingly, 'Is this the Northern Surgical Leviathan, the crack lithotomist, the founder of a "maison de santé", the publisher of "Reports" (with half the facts omitted)?'

The comments were unjust for the work which Syme did at Minto House represented a considerable advance in surgery and he embodied all this experience in the text-books he published. Syme need not be criticised for his publicity methods for they were acceptable at the time and the common practice of the London surgeons. He had undoubtedly a sense of mission in his active propagation of surgical knowledge. If he could be faulted it was for his unfortunate style of writing which to many made it appear that he was always right, that he was above criticism and that the opinions of others were valueless. The London critics reflected resentment that a provincial should presume to dictate to them. The Edinburgh critics were usually motivated by jealousy, particularly those who worked in the Infirmary.[33]

In 1831 Syme published his *Principles of Surgery* which received favourable reviews and was quickly established as a standard work, even in London. It was reprinted the next year and went into many further editions. In this book Syme presented his complete course of lectures covering the basic principles of surgery. The writing is clear and economical but the style is dull with little enlivenment by case details from personal experience. While dogmatic with regard to treatment there are references to the work of others in the discussion of pathology which reveal that the author had read widely in ancient and contemporary literature. As a sound, solid text-book for the student it gave a complete review of surgical theory and practice and was superior to other contemporary works in which vague theories were often accepted without question.

47

More important was Syme's publication in the same year of a *Treatise on the Excision of Diseased Joints*. Tuberculous disease of the major joints was extremely common in the nineteenth century and until Syme put forward his views the usual treatment of the more advanced conditions was by amputation which carried a risk of death in at least one case out of three. Influenced by the work of Park of Liverpool and Crampton of Dublin, Syme developed the conservative procedure by which the diseased joint tissues were removed with preservation of a limb which functioned reasonably well. He favoured this joint excision particularly for the elbow and its advocacy for the knee by other surgeons involved him for many years in bitter argument. His results for the elbow joint were remarkable for of 14 patients only 2 died, this without antisepsis or anaesthesia. In retrospect it was said of Syme in relation to his work on the excision of joints 'if he had done nothing else, he would have been one of the benefactors of the human race'.

Syme by his energy and determination had quickly established himself in surgery. His further advancement and the fulfilment of his ambition to be a leader in his profession could be achieved only by an increase of his influence in the College of Surgeons and in the University. In 1829 he had ousted Robert Knox from the post of Curator of the College Museum. At this time Knox's reputation had suffered a decline as the result of the Burke and Hare scandal and when Syme had rather a trivial quarrel with Knox over the preparation of a specimen the College was only too willing to appoint him in Knox's place. There was a larger issue when in 1831 William Turner was translated from the Chair of Surgery in the College to a University Chair of Surgery. Syme must have been interested in the University appointment but it does not seem that his candidature went forward, perhaps because of the jealousy of the Infirmary staff towards him. He applied for the College Chair with considerable hope of success. His main rival was John Lizars and the election took place in October 1832. There were two factions and prominent in that against Syme was Liston. On the first count there were 23 votes for Lizars and 22 for Syme, with 14 abstentions. Syme's supporters insisted that the votes should

48

be scrutinised and invoked a law that any Fellow more than £2 in debt to the College could not vote. As it turned out this did not help Syme because one of his supporters was thus made ineligible and the final count was 23–21 in favour of Lizars. The result was distressing, if not infuriating, to Syme and it triggered off an antagonism to Lizars which lead to a series of unsavoury quarrels and litigations from which neither derived any credit. In this personal vendetta Syme was revealed in his most vindictive and unforgiving character. Syme's career and reputation were more than once threatened by such controversies and from his handling of these incidents there are insights into his character. It is relevant to digress to describe briefly his arch-enemy Lizars.[34]

John Lizars (1794–1860) after serving for several years in the navy settled in Edinburgh. He had qualified there in 1809 after being apprentice to John Bell. He became a successful extra-mural teacher in surgery and anatomy. He was the first in Great Britain to remove an ovarian tumour successfully and he pioneered other formidable operations such as ligature of the innominate artery and removal of the jaw. He published many books including his magnificent atlases of anatomical plates, skilfully engraved by his brother William Lizars. There were scathing criticisms by some of his rivals such as Robert Knox, who referred to them as 'huge misrepresentations of nature', but they fulfilled an essential need at a time when opportunities for dissection were limited. Despite his many achievements Lizars never won real fame or success. He was a short, stout man whose benign appearance belied his pugnacious and perverse character. His temper ruined his prospects of advancement and limited his success in private practice so that he died in poverty. It was written of him by a contemporary 'he is not very popular with some of his professional brethren. . . . He is too free, blunt and natural.' Somehow or other he always ran into trouble, he was excessively sensitive to criticism and his peppery temper led him to attack others in a manner which often laid him open to litigation. He quarrelled with his colleagues, with institutions, with the powerful editors of the journals and with the government. He became, in particular, the opponent of Liston and of Syme. To them he was the rival for the domination of surgical practice in Edinburgh. In his public quarrels with Syme, Lizars came out the worse of the two but on the whole he was treated unjustly. He deserves to occupy a higher place than is at present accorded to him in surgical history. His eclipse illustrates very clearly how at this time a man's career was often ruined by the jealousies and ruthless criticisms of his colleagues.[35]

Syme had not long to wait before something more important came his way. James Russell had been appointed Professor of Clinical Surgery in 1803 and, as has already been noted, was in the curious position of teaching a clinical subject without the advantage of having his own beds in the Infirmary. He was now 78 and his powers were declining. Like Monro *tertius* he had outlived his age and he still wore the knee breeches and black silk stockings of earlier days. By a curious arrangement Russell was entitled to be paid compensation if he resigned his life appointment and so he demanded that his successor should provide him with an annuity for his retirement. As this was a Crown appointment political influence was involved but little is known of the machinations of the interested parties. Liston, then firmly established in Edinburgh as an able if cantankerous surgeon, was Syme's main rival for the post. Liston offered his candidature to Lord Melbourne and is said to have expressed the view that there should be no question of paying an annuity to Russell. Liston was told that this was perfectly legal and in 1833 Syme was appointed accepting that he should pay Russell £300 a year as long as he survived. It did not cost Syme too much for Russell died three years later!

Syme's appointment started off the usual accusations and misrepresentations. A correspondent, who had some personal animosity towards him, wrote in the *Lancet* that he had 'bought his situation instead of gaining it by talent'. Liston repeatedly affirmed that the whole affair was a piece of disgraceful connivance on the part of the government and that Syme had arranged to pay Russell after secret negotiations with him. Such attacks which persisted for many years were not justified for Syme had certainly proved his ability and in 'purchasing' the Chair he was merely conforming to an accepted custom which was applicable to many other such appointments.

Liston must have resented the success of his former pupil and in 1835 he left Edinburgh to become Professor of Surgery in the newly established University College of London. There he quickly established himself as a leading surgeon and when the causes of rivalry subsided there was a partial reconciliation, albeit rather grudging on the part of Syme. With Liston in London the field was clear for Syme to dominate Edinburgh.

On his transfer to this higher sphere Syme was able to negotiate an appointment to the Infirmary where as an assistant surgeon he was allowed 30 beds. The Commission relating to his appointment stated that he had 'full power to examine candidates and do everything which may be required and necessary to the graduation of Doctors of Medicine'. The Town Council, whose members did not very much like the fact that the Crown had powers to appoint some of the professors, thought that this sentence gave Syme rather sweeping powers. However, on April 6th one of the magistrates introduced Syme to the Senate. His position was a delicate one for it was further stipulated: [36]

> that the professors of medicine, anatomy and surgery shall not by the present appointment be deprived of giving clinical lectures on surgery in the Royal Infirmary and that the said James Syme shall not deliver a course of lectures there at the same time with the Professors of Medicine, Anatomy and Surgery—secondly, that the lectures to be delivered by the said James Syme shall not upon any pretence whatever be converted into a general course of lectures on Anatomy or on the Practice of Surgery, but shall consist of remarks on Cases falling immediately under his own observation.

He was appointed for life with a salary of £100 a year. There was some argument about his share of the students' fees but any financial problems were offset by the fact that he now had a position of great influence. Opportunities for teaching and for pursuing his particular interests in surgery were now increased. He was rapidly becoming the foremost surgeon in Scotland and he had no hesitation in challenging his London colleagues as a leader. His private practice increased and henceforth he lived in comfortable circumstances. His financial independence was further assured by the arrival of a rich and eccentric uncle from India who insisted that his nephew should care for him in his failing health and when he died he left Syme half of a considerable fortune.

Syme had been a professor for seven years before Simpson joined him on the Senate. If anything Simpson's career had been even more meteoric. Within five years of being recognised as a specialist in obstetrics he presented himself as a candidate for the Chair of Midwifery, vacated by Hamilton in 1839. He was only 28 and although professorial appointments were not unusual at an even younger age there was a feeling that here was something wrong about a young man, unmarried at that, attaining such a highly responsible position concerned with the teaching of such a delicate subject. Simpson had undoubtedly held the ambition to succeed Hamilton for a long time and in a very few years he had equipped himself for the job remarkably well. More is known of this election than of Syme's and the story has its drama and throws light on the way in which these things were done.

In 1839, although established as far as his teaching and clinical reputation were concerned, Simpson was in constant financial difficulties. As yet he had not acquired much private practice. However, with the help of his ever willing brothers he had bought the two essentials for a consultant, his own house and his own carriage. The appearance of prosperity suggested by his occupation of 2 Dean Terrace was rather illusory but his financial risks were calculated and perhaps reasonable in his circumstances. Granted good health he was confident that he would succeed and he had the character and strength of will to do so.

On November 15th 1839, he sent in his application. The patronage was in the hands of the Lord Provost, Magistrates and Council. If influence was to be effective it had to be exerted locally. Unlike a Crown appointment the Government of the day had no direct interest. While some of the members of the Council might lend an ear to the advice of influential outsiders they were, in general, an independent body and flattered themselves that they knew how to select the right man. Just how the worthy tradesmen, who largely comprised the Council, were expected to assess the technical and scientific abilities of five aspiring obstetricians is not quite clear. From the start it was certain that the contest would be close and that inevitably there would be bitterness and unpleasantness. Aware of all this Simpson threw himself into the fray with his usual energy. He had to depend mainly on making his case directly to the Council by producing evidence of exceptional ability and experience in the field of obstetrics. It was considered essential to collect a multitude of testimonials. This custom was regarded by many with suspicion but there was no escape from conforming to it. While the election was in progress the *Lancet* reported scornfully 'Every post in London and Dublin carries urgent prayers for testimonials. "Send us testimonials" and he who can produce in his favour the largest batch of fulsome lies under his name is to win the Chair.'

Simpson produced about 70 testimonials. The originals can still be seen and they must have been rather bewildering to the Council. While support from such well known men as Sharpey, Thomson and Reid of Edinburgh, from Crampton and Montgomery of Dublin and from Rigby and Locock of London might have meant something to the Council it is difficult to see what they made of the numerous French and German letters, although perhaps these were translated for them. Some of the letters were flattering and could be helpful but many referred only to a cursory knowledge of Simpson's writings. Rather surprisingly there was a letter from Robert Lee of London who was, initially at least, a candidate himself! Even more surprising Lee seemed to think that Simpson was applying for the Chair in Aberdeen! Perhaps the sheer volume of the testimonials impressed the selection committee and there is evidence that for similar appointments the Council were rather hypnotised by letters from foreign professors. It was an expensive business for Simpson as the printing of this volume of letters cost no less than £168 2s. 1d.![37]

Testimonials were not enough and Simpson had to wield all the pressure he could on individual members of the Council either directly or through his many powerful friends. We know, for example, that he got Mr Walter Grindlay of

Liverpool to write to John Hope, Solicitor-General of Scotland, seeking his support. Hope sent a reply to Grindlay with
a firm rebuff. He did not believe that the Council: [38]

> would appoint a young man however promising his talents
> . . . he is very inexperienced as a canvasser and in disappoint-
> ment at my answer he stated that your political vengeance
> would be the consequence. I reserve my advice to him on this
> subject till after the present stir he may be able to profit by
> them. He came to me too much as claiming a right. This did
> not of course influence my answer previously to his brother
> John. It would have given me very great pleasure had either
> my knowledge of Dr Simpson's acquirements or my connection
> with any of the patrons enabled me to forward your wishes.
> It would have been but a small return for the long journey
> you took from Liverpool to the Linlithgow Poll in June 1838
> and for your kind support.

The letter is interesting because it shows the immaturity
of Simpson in his tactless canvassing: it shows how his
family were deeply involved in the election campaign: it
shows also the political undercurrents. Just how important
Hope's support would have been is uncertain but there was
help from other quarters.

The other candidates were Kennedy, Campbell, Renton
and Thatcher. Robert Lee, a well known but eccentric obstetrician from London, had withdrawn. Thatcher was an
established teacher of some repute in Edinburgh, Simpson
in fact had studied under him. The main rival, however, was
Kennedy of Dublin who had more experience than Simpson,
was older and was better known in the obstetric world.
Simpson's advantage was that he was an Edinburgh man and
known personally to many members of the Council. Some
of the more canny members were, however, afraid that he
would not attract rich patients to the city as Hamilton had
done, to the benefit of the local shop-keepers and hoteliers!
(They were soon to learn how wrong they were about this.)
Simpson's disadvantages were his youth, his unmarried state
and his lowly origin. While the university professors were
not directly involved in the election it is significant that
Simpson wrote to Mr Grindlay on January 22nd indicating
that some of the Senate were in great dread that a 'poor

baker's son' would be elected. Nevertheless he remained confident at this stage that he had a chance of winning.

Although he could not add to his years he could eliminate at least one objection, his unmarried state. For several years he had maintained an increasingly affectionate correspondence with Jessie Grindlay and had become engaged to her in November 1839. He wrote to Mr Grindlay before the end of the year: [39]

> In asking your daughter's hand I ask it, not with any certainty of being elected, and thus having a future at once at my feet —I ask it for better or worse, whether I succeed or, what is more probably, do not succeed. But taking it at the worse I do think by my practice alone to maintain a wife respectably. At the same time I am sure you will pardon me if I tell you —indeed it is my bounden duty to tell you—that, as I stand just now, I am in debt.

Mr Grindlay must have had complete faith in him and certainly Jessie was ready to marry at short notice. In the midst of the turmoil of the canvass Simpson went hurriedly to Liverpool and there on the 26th December married Jessie Grindlay. There was no honeymoon as the election campaign was at its most crucial point and back they went to Edinburgh.

Mrs Simpson was immediately pressed into helping with the preparation of the catalogue of her husband's museum. One of the essentials for a candidate was that he should possess his own collection of specimens and other teaching material and Kennedy had stolen a march by having already published his catalogue. Simpson, however, soon had printed a 'List of the preparations, casts, drawings, instruments, obstetric machinery etc. contained in Dr J. Y. Simpson's Museum and employed by him in the illustration of his lectures on midwifery'. In the foreword he apologised for the hurried manner in which it had been drawn up. He listed some 700 items including plaster casts, oil paintings, osteological preparations, bottled monstrosities and statistical tables. The 'obstetric machinery' was a series of leather models of foetuses and bony pelves used in demonstrating manoeuvres of obstetrics. The instruments included Smellie's original obstetric forceps. It must have cost Simpson a lot to acquire all this paraphernalia and the printing of the catalogue was yet another item to increase his debts.[40]

Three days before the election he wrote to his mother-in-law who seems to have given some financial help at this stage:[41]

This horrid canvass had almost completely emptied our purse and Jessie and I were beginning altogether to lose heart when your kindness—your great kindness restored it.

. . . the canvass stands thus. There are thirty-three voters and I have secured fifteen.

Jessie and I were up at four this morning writing the last part of a catalogue of my museum.

Up to the last minute the general opinion was that Kennedy would be elected by a small margin. The rumour got around that he was a poor lecturer and his supporters hastily brought him to Edinburgh to prove otherwise. His performance did not greatly enhance his reputation. There were political undercurrents and it was suggested by some that the Whigs wanted Simpson to succeed only to keep him out of another appointment.

On Tuesday, 4th February 1840, the result was announced and Simpson wrote to his mother-in-law:[42]

Jessie's honeymoon and mine is to begin tomorrow. I was elected Professor today by a MAJORITY OF ONE. Hurrah!!!

To his father-in-law he wrote:

I was this day elected *Professor*. My opponent had 16—and I had 17 votes. All the *political* influence of both the leading Whigs and Tories there was employed against me—but never mind—I have got the Chair in despite of them—Professors and all—Jessie and Mina send their kindest love. Jessie's honeymoon and mine is to commence tomorrow.

The students cheered when they heard the result. Congratulations flowed in from all quarters but the triumph was appreciated most of all by his own family. His sister Mary, who had been as a second mother to him, heard the glad news as she sailed for Tasmania and at once wrote to him expressing her delight. The faithful brothers now had the reward of their unstinting support over the years. The power of the Town Council to elect professors had often been criticised and sometimes abused but this time the members could well flatter themselves on their perspicacity.

Simpson was now in a position to enhance his reputation and could look forward to a greatly increasing private practice. Even although his commission indicated that he would receive 'no Fee or Salary from the City' he could count on a share of students' fees. There were, however, clouds on the horizon. The supporters of Kennedy were disgruntled and there was a strong faction on the Senate who resented Simpson's appointment. Simpson may have exaggerated what appeared to him a hostile attitude based on his humble origin. He was young and inexperienced when he found himself thrown into the intrigues of the University and it would have served him better if at first he had remained neutral in such delicate matters as the appointment of new professors. Very soon he was writing to Mr Grindlay, 'I have been battling with my brother professors since I came home in order to support the dignity of my Chair and I hope have sufficiently shown them that I am their equal in professional rank.' As Professor of Midwifery (his full title in his Commission was Professor of Medicine and Midwifery and of the Diseases of Women and Children) he was bound to encounter opposition from those who held chairs which had been established much earlier. He may have been over-sensitive to the attitudes of some of his colleagues because he was so much younger and he certainly had a strong feeling that many regarded him as socially and intellectually their inferior.

Syme was amongst those who were reluctant to accept Simpson as an equal. Syme did his best to have Kennedy appointed and Simpson resented that in a testimonial for Kennedy, Syme had written that 'out of all question' Kennedy should be elected. Simpson thought this phrase savoured of deliberate contempt for him but the words seem in their context perfectly reasonable and it is difficult to agree with the rather sanctimonious Duns who regarded the phrase as quite unforgivable 'even for a purely Christian man'! When Simpson was chosen Syme wrote to Sharpey 'I hope you may be right about Simpson but much fear etc. etc. He shall have a fair trial and nothing will give me more pleasure than his turning out better than expected.' One would like to know if 'etc. etc.' was expurgated from the letter or if Syme had already expressed adverse views about Simpson and did not need to repeat them to his friend Sharpey. The fragment of the letter at least hints at the beginning of trouble.[43]

CHAPTER 5

The Rival Professors (1840-1850)

ETWEEN 1840 and 1850 Syme and Simpson became
deeply involved in university affairs, both contributed
widely to their specialties and both were tempted to
quit the Edinburgh scene. For Simpson the decade was made
memorable by his discovery of the use of chloroform and his
work on anaesthesia demands a full record in a separate
chapter. Some unhappy affairs disturbed the smooth progress
of their careers. Whether such quarrels advanced the causes
for which they fought or arrested progress is not easy to decide.

In 1840 Syme was engaged in a litigation with Lizars which
originated in a typically thoughtless piece of writing on the
part of the latter. In his 'System of Practical Surgery', published in 1838, Lizars in a discussion of the treatment of
fistula embellished his text with the following remarks: [44]

> Another case came under the care of our Professor of Clinical
> Surgery who . . . left the part inadequately defended and
> dreadful haemorrhage ensued . . . the Professor was sent for,
> arrived, groped about . . . with his knife, searching for a
> needle in a hayrick—I mean for a blood vessel to be tied:
> meantime the life of the patient was saved by deliquium
> animi: but to this day the wound remains infected and the
> unfortunate man a miserable invalid. . . .

Syme was furious and at once brought a case against Lizars
for a false and calumnious statement calculated to injure
his reputation. The defence had to admit at the last minute
that although Syme had first operated on the patient, it was
an assistant who had dealt so ineffectually with the complication of bleeding. Lizars maintained that he had quoted the
episode only to emphasise the dangers of the particular opera-

59

tion and that, in any case, Syme quite often criticised other surgeons in *his* writings. Lizars had been told that if an apology was forthcoming the case would be dropped but he was too hot-headed to retract. Various doctors came forward to testify that Syme had been slandered. The judge deplored the whole business and criticised the sensitivity and jealousy of the medical profession. Syme won the case and was awarded £50—rather less than the £1,000 damages which were sought.[45]

Compared with much that was written in the London journals of the time the slander was mild. Lizars as usual had got some of his facts wrong and this went against him. The feud which had simmered since the election in the College was now increasingly bitter. There was one argument after another, usually in the correspondence columns of the journals. For example when Syme implied in an article that he alone was successful in the operative treatment of popliteal aneurysm and all others in Edinburgh had failed, Lizars wrote rather plaintively, 'Professor Syme shows his zeal for the improvement of surgery at the expense of much illiberality towards his professional brethren. . . .'

In the University there were many controversial issues particularly in relation to professional appointments. The Chair of Pathology held by Thomson was the subject of an acrimonious discussion in which Syme and Simpson were in direct opposition. In 1837 Syme had started a campaign against the continuance of the teaching of pathology as a separate subject and had stated that 'general pathology is not only useless but injurious': Syme believed that pathology was best taught by the clinician dealing with a particular branch of medicine or surgery but it may be conjectured that he and his supporters were exceedingly jealous of letting any branch of teaching out of their hands. Syme despised the specialisation in pathology which had permeated some European schools but which was so far generally unaccepted in Great Britain. Simpson, on the other hand, had a much broader outlook and he entered the fray to support the teaching of pathology as a separate subject with great conviction and energy. He had taught pathology when he acted as a deputy to Professor Thomson and he recognised that as

60

medical science advanced it was necessary to sub-divide the branches and to increase the number of teachers. His arguments were put forward in a masterly manner and he issued a pamphlet which swept aside the case which Syme had advanced in his rather narrow-minded effusions. It was a tribute to Simpson's force of character and his clear exposition of the subject that he, a very junior professor, carried the day against more powerful and well-established colleagues such as Syme and Alison. He had been feeling his way up to this time and his success in this particular battle established his confidence and his influence in University matters. It was perhaps a little unfortunate that William Henderson (1810–1872) was chosen as the new Professor of Pathology for he quite soon professed homoeopathy and by doing so involved the Edinburgh school in much trouble.[46]

In 1842 Charles Bell died while holding the Chair of Surgery in which he had succeeded Turner. He had come back to Edinburgh from London in 1836 and had been appointed almost unanimously for his notable achievements in surgery and anatomy. The fancied candidates were John Lizars, Robert Knox and James Miller. Knox although a brilliant anatomist had not lived down his involvement in the Burke and Hare case and in any case in his numerous applications for similar positions he ruined his chance by scorning to provide testimonials, wrung, as he put it, 'from polite foreigners . . . disgraceful documents, stalking horses under covert of which the foulest jobs have been perpetrated.' He was rather prone to slander his opponents during these elections and to castigate the patrons. He soon ruined his chances for this chair as he had for many others in the past.

There is no direct evidence that Simpson was a close friend of Lizars but he might have been influenced by the fact that Syme would inevitably be against his surgical rival. Simpson did not behave in a very gentlemanly fashion as far as Miller was concerned. He did an unforgiveable thing by bringing up from past history the story of an operation done by Miller in which disaster had followed. In 1835 Miller saw a patient, in consultation with Simpson, with an orbital aneurysm and, as was the recognised practice, he ligatured the carotid artery. The patient died and Simpson did an autopsy to find that the vagus nerve had been included in the arterial ligature. Miller was aware of the autopsy findings but he published the case without mentioning the accident. Simpson opposed Miller on the grounds that he had been professionally dishonest. Simpson at least came out into the open to attack Miller but Syme was even more ungentlemanly for he sent an anonymous letter to the patrons condemning Miller for the same reasons. Despite these attacks Miller was elected. Syme and Miller remained on uneasy terms and at times had bitter quarrels. Simpson and Miller became near neighbours in Queen Street, they were united in their support of the Free Church at the time of the Disruption and they collaborated in the first clinical trials of chloroform. Nevertheless they fluctuated between friendship and antagonism.[47]

These were quarrels at University level but in everyday practice similar outbursts of jealousy, temper and bad manners were not unusual. In 1845 Syme wrote to Beilby, the President of the College of Physicians, complaining of Simpson's unprofessional behaviour. By this time Syme resented Simpson's incursions into fields which he thought were outside the scope of a physician-accoucheur. Syme had referred in an article to the mismanagement of a case by Simpson. The whole affair was blown up into exaggerated importance by the intrigues of Dr Cormack, the editor of the journal concerned. The quarrel was not resolved by tactful discussion or by an exchange of letters but instead it came to a head almost as a brawl on the landing in a patient's house. Syme had been called by Beilby to see a case and when he emerged on the staircase he met Simpson on a similar errand. Quivering with rage and within earshot of their patient the two distinguished consultants indulged in a violent argument with Simpson accusing Syme of publishing defamatory statements. The story of this unruly scene reached even London and William Fergusson wrote to Simpson expressing gratification 'by the manner in which you have kept a certain old friend of mine in proper order, no one, since I left, having had the courage to do so but yourself.' Things between them reached such a pitch that Simpson announced that he would in future avoid Syme's professional company. Simpson contemplated a litigation but for a fee of 6s. 8d. Robertson, his solicitor, advised him against pursuing the matter.[48]

Despite this disturbing background to their lives both men were meanwhile achieving much that was constructive and bringing advances to medical science. Syme, after he was appointed professor, continued to publish clinical reports in the *Edinburgh Journal* recording all his wide experience and methodically impressing his views on the theory and practice of surgery. His work continued on aneurysms, on joint excisions, on the removal of tumours of the jaw, on lithotomy and the countless other subjects which are listed in the bibliography appended to this volume. He was like all surgeons of the time particularly interested in amputations and had been largely concerned in introducing in Great Britain the flaps method by which the stump was covered with skin and healed much better than did the exposed stump after the old circular incision. In 1843 he perfected the amputation at the ankle joint still known by his name. In his time this was an ingenious and useful procedure as artificial limbs were crude and the preservation of the whole length of the leg with a stump which could tolerate weight-bearing was of great practical value. Although today the method is seldom applicable, for 100 years it had a very useful place.

While Syme in all these publications announced no great new discovery, he established by his sound reasoning many procedures originated by others. He was not, however, very ready to try out revolutionary techniques. In 1845 Richard Oliver reported in the *Edinburgh Journal* the successful transfusion of 22 ounces of blood to a woman with severe uterine bleeding. This was one of many sporadic reports on the possibilities of blood transfusion. Syme dismissed the procedure as impracticable on the grounds that cases for which it was suggested were usually hopeless from other aspects. Rather weakly he affirmed that if transfusion was urgently needed for sudden blood loss there would not be time to get the apparatus together. His attitude, as usual, was essentially practical but he showed little imagination in discussing this kind of problem. He scorned, rightly, vague theories about transfusion such as that expounded by Lizars at this time who advocated an almost homoeopathic dose of one or two drachms, affirming that this 're-excites the heart and puts the strings of life into action'.

His *Principles of Surgery* went into successive editions and retained its popularity although some reviewers described it as 'too parochial'. In 1838 he had published a monograph on *Diseases of the Rectum*. This dealt almost entirely with the minor but important conditions such as fistula. Syme was never one to prophesy advances in surgery and he dismissed the suggestion, already current, that malignant tumours of the rectum might be removed surgically. Of this idea he wrote, 'an operation so dreadful in its performance and effects, as cutting out the end of the bowel, together with its sphincter, is to be deeply regretted, as well for the credit of surgery as the good of humanity'.

In 1848 there appeared his *Contributions to the Pathology and Practice of Surgery*. This was rather a hotch-potch of his previous writings and was possibly produced to boost his reputation in London, for it was in this year he went to University College Hospital. Syme included his short paper on the solution of rubber which, as it hardly had to do with surgery, must have been inserted as a reminder that *he* had invented the waterproofing process and not Macintosh! While some of the papers reproduced were important Syme paid the penalty for this scrappy collection in a cold reception from the critics. The *British and Foreign Medico-Chirurgical Review* wrote: [49]

> We find little in the remaining papers to interest or detain us . . . we must confess our sincere regret that we have been unable to bestow unqualified praise . . . bound to notice the egotistical tone of the writer and his almost contemptuous reference to the opinions and practice of his contemporaries. Mr Syme never loses an opportunity of telling us that he was the first to suggest some new plan of treatment. . . .

Such criticisms were to some extent just but in 1848 there were factions in London exceedingly jealous of his influence. To some his subsequent election to the Chair of Surgery in University College Hospital was anathema and to others it was even worse that, having got the Chair, he should have dared to give it up!

Syme had proved himself an able teacher in his Minto House days. He relied on two methods to impart instruction to his students. His lectures, although delivered in a low voice, commanded absolute attention. That his students absorbed every detail is shown in the notes which still survive. Beveridge, for example, wrote up in a series of six manuscript books Syme's full course of lectures and from these we learn that in the winter and spring terms of 1852–53 Syme covered the whole of surgery in 120 lectures. The clarity of these and other records speak for the intense care with which Syme prepared his lectures. More original was Syme's method of clinical teaching. He detested the London method by which a group of students followed their chief round the ward, and relied on chance remarks and mutterings when they stopped at each bed. Syme believed that this method was unpleasant for the patient and that it did not allow free discussion. He preferred to bring a selected patient into the lecture room and that first of all the dresser in charge should give the history of the case. Syme would then draw attention to the more obvious signs and symptoms showing the simple things which could be observed by all. He dismissed the patient and gave a full discussion of the problems of diagnosis and management. He brought this technique to a fine art and was convinced that this was the best way to inculcate basic surgical principles. If an operation was done the theatre was large enough to accommodate the surgery class and the visitors who thronged to Edinburgh to see Syme at work. It was evidence of his unique skill as a teacher that in his audience there would be many of his old pupils in practice in Edinburgh, or even from further afield, avid to learn more from their master. There was a ritual about it all and of many eye-witness accounts that by Joseph Bell is one of the most vivid. The theatre was soon filled when an important operation was posted up: [50]

Chairs in the arena were kept for colleagues or distinguished strangers; first row for dressers on duty: operating table in centre: Mr Syme on a chair in left centre . . . a meek little wooden chair without arms. House surgeon a little behind, but nearer the door: instrument clerk with his well stocked table under the big window. He comes in, sits down with a little, a very little, bob of a bow, rubs his trouser legs with both hands open and signs for the first case. The four dressers on duty and in aprons, march in (if possible in step) carrying a rude wicker basket, in which, covered by a rough red blanket the patient peers up at the great amphitheatre crammed with faces. A brief description . . . then the little, neat, round shouldered, dapper man takes his knife and begins: and the merest tyro sees at once a master of his craft at work—no show, little elegance, but absolute certainty, ease and determination: rarely a word to an assistant—they should know their business if the unexpected happens . . . the patient is sent off . . . and then comes a brief commentary, short, sharp and decisive, worth taking down verbatim, if you can manage it, yet he has no notes, a very little veiled voice, and no eloquence. The discipline of the class is perfect, even the idlers are shamed and interested into quietness.

Simpson too was recording a mass of important work in relation to his specialty and touching also on subjects of wider interest in medicine or surgery. From 1838 he sent to the *Edinburgh Journal* a series of 'Contributions to Intraperitoneal pathology' and to the Edinburgh Obstetrical Society, of which he was President from 1841 to 1857, he read many papers. When we add the articles he wrote in this period for the London and Edinburgh journals the volume of work represented is almost unbelievable. He covered the whole field of obstetrics and gynaecology and introduced many new ideas. In the diagnosis of gynaecological conditions he was a strong advocate of the use of the uterine sound and of the speculum. At the time there was a strong faction against the employment of such instruments and it was greatly due to Simpson that the almost hysterical rejection of such diagnostic aids by many surgeons was counteracted. In the treatment of abnormal labour he advanced new methods, particularly for cases of malposition of the placenta. His theories with regard to the complication of bleeding in the latter type of case were wrong but his practical management was superior to that of his colleagues. In 1840 he advocated and practised an operation for excision of cancer of the uterus, a condition previously treated by local applications of caustics or by the cautery. Syme attacked him for this as he considered that such operative procedures were not in his province. Very little of what he wrote escaped criticism, either to deny the efficacy of a method or to dispute priority in its discovery. His most prominent opponents were the London obstetricians Lee and Tyler-Smith and there was an anonymous correspondent 'I. Irons' (who might have been either Lee or Tyler-Smith). With these rivals and others there were violent slanging matches in the pages of the journals. Some of the criticisms were sound and the arguments did good but often these disputes sank to trivialities or personal abuse and the main issue was forgotten.

Simpson's inventive faculty is well illustrated by his work on the 'air-tractor'. As a substitute for forceps as a means of traction in difficult childbirth, Simpson applied to the on-coming foetal head a 'sucker' device which worked on a very simple principle. As a child he had probably played, as small boys still do, with a sucker of wet leather attached to a string and used it to lift large stones. He applied this simple atmospheric pressure device more elaborately by evacuating air from the space between the child's scalp and the sucker device with a brass pump. He gave a dramatic demonstration of the apparatus at an obstetrical society meeting and showed precisely what force could be exerted. In planning the instrument he went to great trouble, even to the extent of studying the mechanism of the suckers of the cuttle fish and other organisms. For a time the technique had some popularity but it was then discarded. It is an interesting comment, however, on the merit of this particular device that it has been revived in a more sophisticated form in recent years. Needless to say the more conservative obstetricians denounced it. Syme wrote scathingly at a later date:[51]

> I have scrupulously avoided any interference with projects relating to other departments of teaching. Thus when it was proposed to accellerate the progress of babies in entering the world by applying sucking pumps to their tender scalps, however much commiserating the helpless victim of an inventive genius I left the matter entirely to my obstetric colleague. . . .

As usual, an argument over technique became one of priority and an accusation was levelled at Simpson. A Dr

Mitchell announced that when he was a student he had followed a suggestion made by Simpson that an air tractor could be devised. Mitchell maintained that *he* described the apparatus in an examination paper and that when the paper was marked his professor stole the idea without acknowledgement! Simpson denied that he had ever seen the paper and in fact he was ready to award priority to Dr Neil Arnott of London who had made the proposal many years earlier, although he had not developed it practically. Despite all counter-claims Simpson must undoubtedly be given the credit for this ingenious invention.[52]

His interests outside his own subject were vast. Anything unusual fascinated him and he delighted in testing established dogma. To appreciate how ably and logically he could demolish a superstition or an established idea it is worth reading his article on the subject 'Are females born co-twins with males sterile?' The paper begins 'It is a popular opinion and I do not know any instance to discountenance it, that if twins be of different sexes the female is sterile.' John Hunter had observed that in black cattle if male and female calves were born the female was imperfect, sterile and known as a free-martin. Simpson confirmed this fact for himself in the Edinburgh slaughter-houses. He knew that, especially in agricultural communities, this rule was applied to human twins and he realised that any girl born as a twin to a male was considered unmarriageable. He did a simple statistical exercise and found that such twins were unproductive in the ratio of 1 : 10. He compared the sterility rate in non-twins in two different towns and again found the ratio of 1 : 10. He even studied the records of the British Peerage to find a ratio of $1 : 6\frac{1}{9}$ in non-twins. Thus he very clearly demolished a preconceived idea and proved that the fruitfulness of a female twin was unimpaired. Professor Chassar Moir has rightly described this paper as a model of clarity and certainly it shows Simpson's ability to marshal facts and to use statistics in a manner which was almost unknown in his time and which is not always achieved today.[53]

His wider interests in the major problem of hospital infection, then a matter of great concern to any thinking clinician, are revealed by the beginning of his studies of what he termed later 'Hospitalism'. In 1847 he conducted a statistical survey on the mortality rate of major amputations throughout the country. This was primarily concerned with the effect of ether on mortality rates but the survey was of a pattern which he used later in other investigations. He sent a proforma to all the major hospitals in the British Isles and from the replies he developed a mass of statistics far more important than those available to one surgeon or one hospital. Once more he revealed himself as an original investigator and broke new ground on the use of statistical methods.[54]

As a teacher he proved stimulating in his set course of lectures. His personality was such that he commanded attention and he prepared his notes with great care. They were embellished by illustrations from his own wide experience and from his intensive knowledge of early and contemporary writings. His classes were crowded and immensely popular for he treated his students 'in a confiding spirit and not as a superior person'. It has been said that the systematic lecture, so popular in the Scottish medical schools, had the effect that 'information was transferred from the notes of the lecturer to the notes of the student without passing through the brains of either'. With Simpson this was far from the case and all confirm 'his wonderful facility for imparting instruction to others' and how by his 'conciseness, clearness and directness he made his *dull subject* fascinatingly interesting.[55]

Of his clinical teaching at the bedside we know less. His life was so busy that it was the individual student who was fortunate enough to accompany him on a case who was likely to benefit most. Some of these students became attached to him as unofficial apprentices on the old system and for periods lodged with him so that they participated in all his work. Thomas Cunningham, a student in 1848, wrote to his brother:[56]

> I have still pleasure in telling you that Professor Simpson and I are very intimate. . . . He took me with him to a case for the purpose of seeing a child which was born the night before—but died: I had to make the post-mortem. . . .

Simpson's attitudes to his students were indicated when in 1842 it fell to him to give the annual graduation address. He exhorted them to go on studying after qualification and to plan their lives so that not a minute was wasted. He admonished that they should not seek advancement by social connections and reminded them that their duties were primarily to their patients. He enlarged, as well he might, on the rules of etiquette and behaviour in the profession and counselled them to 'live peaceably with all men'. He ended by warning against some of the temptations of life and pleading that they should 'pursue earnestly and undeviatingly the direct course of Christian and professional duty'.[57]

From 1840 onwards Simpson's private work increased rapidly. He took a naïve pleasure in his increasing practice amongst the aristocracy. To his brother he wrote in 1840, 'I saw yesterday one Viscountess and three "Ladies". Good for one day among the nobility.' In 1844 the Princess Marie of Baden, wife of the Duke of Hamilton, came under his care while she was at Holyrood Palace and he wrote, 'I have been exceedingly fortunate in getting the Princess as a patient, because it quietly places me at the top of the *practice* on this side of the Tweed'. Again he wrote, 'In November I expect to bring into the world heirs to the Earldoms of W, R. and M. Of course I calculate on the three youngsters being all boys.' Success in practice amongst the higher levels of society gave him great pleasure but he regarded this not in terms of calculated social climbing but as a fascinating interlude in his experience of humanity. He never forgot his own humble origin and remained the same to rich and poor. The only trouble was that with his rapidly expanding practice appointments were often missed, letters were unanswered and there were many who were ready to criticise him for carelessness and even malpractice. Soon his income increased and some of his debts could at last be paid. A complete financial security eluded him for long owing to his carelessness with money (he once stopped a rattling window with a £5 note he had in his pocket) and his gullibility with regard to investments and speculations.

By 1845 both Syme and Simpson were not only at the head of their specialties in the whole of Scotland but patients were beginning to come north from England. Syme had been appointed Surgeon to the Queen in Scotland in 1837 and

Simpson was made one of Her Majesty's Physicians for Scotland in 1847. These marks of Royal favour counted for much both in Edinburgh and in London. In both there must have been, although in varying degree, the urge to seek further fame in the capital. London was a magnet to Scotsmen, particularly to those in the medical profession. Sir Charles Bell who had left Edinburgh to gain fame in London had written: [58]

> No man unless he had held a high reputation here can fully conceive the gratification attending practice in London . . . an eminent surgeon is received by the first people in a manner most flattering and which I fear, obtains nowhere else. . . . Yestreen I sat between the Chancellor of the Exchequer, the Vice-Chancellor, Sir H. Halford. Can you place me so in Auld Reekie?

Both Syme and Simpson were ambitious men and the opportunities offered in London for professional and social advancement were not to be dismissed lightly. As things turned out Simpson only toyed with the idea while Syme, who perhaps had more to gain, took the plunge but as will be told, his sojourn in London was soon cut short.

Robert Liston had held the Chair of Surgery in the University College Hospital for 12 years and established himself in London with great success. His health was failing when he visited Edinburgh in 1847. During his stay he saw much of Syme with whom the old quarrels were now resolved. He died suddenly and quite unexpectedly in 1847 from a ruptured aneurysm. At short notice his post was offered to Syme. Although now so well established in Edinburgh, not only professionally but also domestically in his fine house and gardens at Millbank, he at once accepted the invitation. Perhaps he had never relinquished an early ambition to seek fame in London, perhaps, although he would scarcely have admitted it, he felt that Simpson with his new prominence from his discovery of chloroform, had rather stolen his thunder. It seems unlikely that he sought for more financial gain but it is certain that he saw in his translation an opportunity to introduce to London his methods of clinical teaching.

Feelings in London were mixed about the appointment. The *Lancet*, up to then a bitter opponent of Syme, did not question his ability but expressed disgust that a London surgeon had not been offered the post and deplored the one-way traffic of doctors from north to south. The affair was regarded as 'a gross piece of Scotch jobbing' on the part of Sharpey, now a professor in University College Hospital. The *Medical Times* regarded the appointment as a strong counter to the nepotism which pervaded almost all of the London hospitals. The students of University College Hospital sent Syme a memorial expressing their pleasure at his appointment.

Edinburgh appreciated that she was to lose one of her foremost leaders. By this time Syme had become an institution and his harsh and uncompromising character was more than compensated for by his undoubted success as surgeon and teacher. Perhaps some of the students who had tolerated ill his stern discipline were not too distressed. Thomas Cunningham, for example, in his letter full of excitement about his contacts with Simpson, stated flatly and without any regret 'Prof. Syme is gone to London, he delivered his last lecture a few days ago. Mr Miller's filling his place at present'. Earlier, in 1842, an 'Edinburgh Student' had written to the *Lancet* about Syme's bad temper with his dressers and how 'students have long suffered from discourteous behaviour of Prof. Syme'.

Nevertheless there was real sorrow at his imminent departure and with Professor Christison in the Chair more than 100 doctors, including many of his old pupils, gathered to honour him at a banquet in February 1848. Simpson did not attend. There were speeches expressing great regret at his resignation and praise of his achievements. Syme expressed his painful feelings on leaving Edinburgh, excused his frequent contributions to the professional turmoil of the city on the grounds of his firm principles and was obviously touched by this demonstration of loyalty from his friends and from most of his colleagues.

He moved at once and purchased a suitable house in Bruton Street, thus quite clearly indicating that he expected to stay in London. In a short time there were problems. He found the students less disciplined than in Edinburgh and was rather appalled at their habit of perching on the iron rails of the lecture theatre instead of being seated in a decorous fashion on benches. But, in general, the students accepted him generously and their behaviour was not the main factor which led to his early resignation. It was the intrigues and mismanagement of the University College Hospital school which worried him. When he took the appointment he understood that he would teach clinical surgery alone and he expected to have time to build up a private practice. He soon found that he was to be inveigled into giving lectures on systematic surgery also and he felt that this would occupy too much of his time. In a statement of his reasons for resigning the position after such a short tenure he gave this as the main cause, but he deplored also the unruly scenes he had witnessed at the Hospital prize-giving when his colleagues, Quain and Sharpey, were submitted to 'contumelious treatment' by the audience. Christison describes the scene as follows: [59]

> The two obnoxious professors were received with groans and vociferations, and prevented from delivering their addresses. . . . No attempt was made by Lord Brougham (the Chancellor) to discourage, or even advise the malcontents. On the contrary when one of the insulted professors made a simple and dignified appeal to his Lordship, he turned it aside by a jocular comparison of the scene before him to what he had witnessed in the House of Commons. . . .
>
> I was present. It is unnecessary to say what were my own sensations. They were lost in observing Mr Syme, who sat among his brother professors, his countenance overspread with an ominous cloud of mingled sorrow and displeasure. . . . Returning home late, he came into the room where I sat reading, paced for some time forward and back again in moody silence, and suddenly stopping in front of me, said, 'I am going back to Edinburgh'.

Syme did not wish to find himself subjected to such insults in future years. As Quain and Sharpey had supported his appointment to University College Hospital he felt that the demonstration was at least indirectly against him. Since he had refused to take on all the duties required of him by the hospital authorities he had no option but to resign. There may have been other reasons, and there were plenty of his enemies who were ready to offer suggestions. Undoubtedly the affairs of University College Hospital were in a parlous state and there were rejected candidates for the post who were ready to make trouble. It was hinted that Syme was disappointed by his reception in London and that, in particular, his expectations of acquiring a large private practice were not realised. He could hardly have expected, however, to build up a new connection in three months! London, on the whole, was not sorry to see him go but it is pleasant to record that the University College Hospital students appreciated him and sent a petition urging him to stay. Syme wrote to a friend with an openness unusual to him: [60]

> . . . how ambition made me sacrifice happiness: how I found such a spirit of dispeace in the College as to forbid any reasonable prospect of comfort: how I resolved to carry into execution the plans for enlarging the house at Millbank and spend the remainder of my days, if I can, as happily as before trying this metropolitan experiment. . . . This is my last day in London and it is impossible to describe the feeling with which we all look forward to our return home.

This and other letters reveal Syme in a more appealing light. The simple fact emerges that he was home-sick!

He sold the house in Bruton Street but the abortive expedition cost him some £2,000. But as he wrote 'I would gladly have paid a larger sum for the peace and comfort of being free from animosity and contention'. Could it be that professional back-biting was even worse in London than in Edinburgh? The whole affair might have been a disaster but this was not so. Millbank had not been sold and he could return to this much loved estate at once. The Managers of the Infirmary had filled Syme's appointment only on a temporary basis and were delighted to restore his wards to him. More important, for some reason, nothing had been done to replace him in the Chair of Clinical Surgery. There was only one difficulty here and that arose from church politics which were active at the time. During Syme's short absence an attempt to invoke the Test Act was in process. Thus a professor in Edinburgh had to belong to the Established Church of Scotland. Syme was then an Episcopalian and could have been rejected on this ground. Somehow he got out of the difficulty and a columnist in one of the contemporary journals suggested that he did so because, although an Episcopalian, he simultan-

eously rented a pew in the established church of St Andrew's!
It is a little difficult to explain how Syme felt justified in
writing to the *Lancet* in June 1848 affirming that he was *not*
an Episcopalian! A new Commission was granted him and
soon he was completely re-instated and in Edinburgh at least
his short absence was soon forgotten. In London the possible
reasons for his resignation continued to provide much material
for the gossip columns.[61]

The temptations and blandishments offered by London
were of less significance to Simpson. By 1847 his discovery of
chloroform had given him international fame while his professional reputation was such that not only did he dominate
obstetric practice in Edinburgh but patients flocked to him
from all over the British Isles. In 1845 he visited London
professionally to undertake the care of a lady of high degree.
He enjoyed his short stay in Stafford House, the residence of
Lord Blantyre, consorted with high society and was agreeably
surprised at his reception. In 1848 when Rigby, one of the
leading obstetricians in London, retired from St Bartholomew's Hospital, feelers were put out as to the possibility of
Simpson accepting the Obstetric Chair. There was a strong
wish that he should do so and the *Lancet* regarded his acceptance as almost a foregone conclusion. The offer came just
after Syme moved to London and it cannot be thought that
Simpson would have wanted to follow him there. More
important were the simple facts that Simpson loved Edinburgh and that he saw no greater opportunity in London
for the expansion of his work and authority than already
existed for him.

About 1843 Syme had moved from his town house in
Charlotte Square and his comfortable income permitted the
purchase of Millbank. This was an elegant house in extensive
grounds and there were greenhouses in which he could indulge in his hobby of cultivating exotic flowers and fruits.
Here he brought up his family, his two daughters by his first
marriage and his son by his second marriage. A few intimate
friends like John Brown were entertained quietly in these
pleasant surroundings. He lived an orderly life, driving at
precisely 10 o'clock to his consulting room in Rutland Street,
visiting his patients in the Infirmary, operating and lectur-

ing to his students. He returned to Millbank for dinner and retired early to his bed. At times he would travel quite far to see patients throughout Scotland and to the North of England but there was no rush and all was done in a carefully planned manner.

Simpson's ménage was more colourful and erratic. An obstetrician's timetable was more liable to disruption but it was his almost manic activity which created conditions which must have at times been the despair of his wife. He soon found that his home in Albany Street was too small for his growing family and his expanding practice. In 1845, for £2,150, he purchased 52 Queen Street, a solid, plain dwelling with the public garden common to the Edinburgh squares and terraces in front of it. Here he spent the remainder of his life, here with his friends he made the trials of chloroform and other anaesthetics and from here he conducted his huge practice. His professional life was carried on at a rollicking pace and Dr Brown described it thus: [62]

> Dr Simpson is well and as overwhelmed with work as ever, and plunging about rejoicing in it, like any seal in the Bay of Baffin.

CHAPTER 6

The Introduction of General Anaesthesia

O N October 16th, 1846, John Warren, surgeon to the
Massachussets General Hospital, did a small operation
on Gilbert Abbot to remove a tumour of the neck.
Abbot was successfully anaesthetised with ether by a dentist
William Morton. The events which preceded this historic
operation are well known although some of the details are
controversial. Before this time alcohol, opium and other drugs
had often been used in attempts to alleviate the pain and
terror of operations but, in general, the surgeon had worked
with the acceptance on his part, and perforce on the part of
the patient, that pain was the inevitable accompaniment of
surgery. We can only wonder at the fortitude of the patient
and at the grim callousness forced upon the surgeon.

In 1800, Humphrey Davy had suggested nitrous oxide
as a means of eliminating pain in surgical procedures but this
idea was not taken up by the medical profession. In 1824,
Henry Hickman of Shifnal, Shropshire, although he produced experimental evidence of the value of carbon dioxide
as an anaesthetic agent, failed to convince other doctors.
Thomas Beddoes (1760-1808), a versatile physician of Bristol,
working in close contact with Davy was more interested in
the therapeutic effects of inhaled gases than in their anaesthetic qualities. The idea of inhalation anaesthesia existed
in the early nineteenth century but its practical application
was retarded. There was a strong feeling, which was to persist
for many years even after the discovery of the anaesthetic
qualities of ether and chloroform, that in some obscure way
pain was a necessary factor which stimulated the resistance
of the patient to the shock of an operation.[63]

In America Davy's observations on the action of nitrous

oxide were investigated further and in 1844, a dentist, Horace Wells, was present when Gardner Collon demonstrated its anaesthetic properties. Wells himself was rendered unconscious by the gas and had a tooth extracted painlessly but his efforts to establish the technique did not convince others. William Morton, also a dentist, was dissatisfied with nitrous oxide and he experimented with sulphuric ether. With the assistance of Charles Jackson, Professor of Chemistry in Boston, Morton used ether successfully for a dental extraction in September 1846. Some of the peculiar effects of the drug were already well known and 'ether frolics' were often indulged in by those seeking excitement or amusement from the intoxicating effects of drinking the pure form. Morton may have been unprincipled in that he sought to patent ether and to retain its formula a secret by colouring it with red dye but he was courageous in that he accepted a challenge from John Warren to demonstrate its use in a surgical operation. The relative claims of Morton and Wells as originators of general anaesthesia remain the subject of much argument and there is a counter-claim on behalf of an American general practitioner Crawford Long, who in 1842 gave ether successfully for a minor surgical operation. The real credit must go to Morton, for it was he who convinced a surgeon in an influential position to use general anaesthesia. Suffice to say that the operation in the Massachussets General Hospital initiated an exciting chain of events.[64]

The repercussions in Great Britain, considering the state of communications at the time, were remarkably quick. The *Liverpool Mercury* of December 18th, 1846 first announced the discovery publicly to England. On November 9th Mr Robinson, surgeon dentist to the London Metropolitan Hospital, acquired a copy of an article by Dr Bigelow in the *Boston Medical and Surgical Journal* describing the use of ether as an anaesthetic. Dr Boott, an American physician practising in London, received the news of ether in a letter from Dr Bigelow on December 17th. With Robinson he devised an inhalation apparatus and on December 19th used it for a dental extraction. Dr Boott wrote at once to Robert Liston who discussed the innovation with his friend Dr Peter Squire. The weekend was spent in experiments and Squire's nephew

William was used as a guinea-pig with encouraging results. On December 21st at University College Hospital, Liston felt justified in using ether for a major operation. The patient was a Harley Street butler, Frederick Churchill, aged 36, and the operation was a thigh amputation for chronic bone infection.[65]

Liston's successful use of ether was well publicised and must remain of great historical importance as it was the first acceptance of ether anaesthesia in England by a surgeon of influence and repute. The scene has been immortalised in a rather inaccurate painting which is often reproduced. This was commissioned 40 years after the event and shows as spectators the young student Joseph Lister and the rising young naval surgeon Thomas Spencer Wells. Wells was not present at the operation as he was serving in Malta at the time. Lister may have been present but this is uncertain as he did not begin his clinical studies until more than a year later.[66]

The letter from Bigelow to Boott came in the fast mail ship *Acadia*. In this there travelled as ship's surgeon William Fraser of Dumfries. He knew about Morton's demonstration of ether anaesthesia and may even have been present at the operation on October 16th. The ship docked at Liverpool on December 16th and Fraser reached his home in Dumfries within three days. This enthusiastic young man told his colleagues at the Dumfries Infirmary of the new discovery and persuaded them to use ether for an accident case which had just been admitted. On December 17th, two days before Liston's operation, general anaesthesia was given at Dumfries for an operation of which the details are uncertain. James McLauchlan, the senior surgeon, was present but it seems likely that the anaesthetic was given by a younger surgeon William Scott and that he having rendered the patient unconscious then performed the operation. The details were corroborated by Scott in 1872 when, 26 years later, he wrote a letter on the subject to the *Lancet*. There is other circumstantial evidence which supports these facts. The priority is not of great importance but in later years Simpson was at pains to claim for Scotland the first use of ether in the British Isles for a major operation.[67]

Returning to Liston's operation it is right to emphasise the part played by Boott, Robinson and the Squires in persuading Liston to use ether and in devising the apparatus. Surprisingly in the numerous reports there is little direct mention of the anaesthetist but it is reasonably certain that this was Dr Peter Squire. Liston had no doubt of the importance of the occasion and it was celebrated at a party at his house the same evening. After dinner, intoxicated by success, Liston and his friends persuaded William Cadge (1822-1903), later to become a distinguished surgeon in Norwich, to submit himself to further tests and he was duly rendered unconscious with ether! The tradition of self-experimentation in anaesthesia was thus established and we must admire the courage, perhaps often verging on foolhardiness, of these pioneers.

Liston's case was reported in the *Medical Times* of December 26th, 1846 very briefly and further particulars were eagerly awaited. On January 2nd, 1847 the *Medical Times* reprinted Bigelow's account of ether anaesthesia from the Boston journal and from King's College Hospital came the reports of a further three successful operations under ether done by William Fergusson. In the same number Robinson wrote to claim priority in using ether successfully in Great Britain for dental extractions and described his apparatus in detail. There was a letter also from James Dorr indicating that he was to act for the American inventors and would protect a patent already taken out in their favour. This raised an outcry and it was greatly deplored that a method directed at the amelioration of human suffering should be so protected. Whatever the legal considerations advanced at the time 'Letheon', as ether was described commercially, was at once freely and readily available to anyone who cared to use it.[68]

Soon all the journals were publishing reports of etherisation in London and in the provinces. The correspondence columns were filled with letters claiming priority for the new discovery. Dr Collyer of Jersey announced that he had given ether to produce insensibility many years earlier 'without the most remote idea of remuneration'. Dr Dudley wrote in support of Hickman as the pioneer quoting Hickman's *Memorial to the King of France* in 1824 on the subject, not perhaps the best medium of propagating medical knowledge! Criticisms there were in plenty. There were moral and theological arguments on the necessity and desirability of pain. Some French reports suggested that sexual passion and excitement were aroused in women and an English correspondent wrote: [69]

> I may venture to say, that to the women of this country the bare possibility of having feelings of such a kind excited and manifested in outward uncontrollable actions, would be more shocking even to anticipate, than the endurance of the last extremity of physical pain.

Victorian gentlemen were ready to spring to the defence of the virtue of wife or daughter but not so ready to relieve her of the pains of labour.

The new discovery was taken up with almost alarming rapidity. Doctors practised on each other and had no hesitation in using ether on their patients despite the scantiest appreciation of its action. Elaborate devices were hastily constructed by modifying various types of inhalation bottles and their respective merits were argued interminably. A note of warning was sounded in the *Medical Times* of March 6th, 1847 when the first two fatal cases were reported. There was an inquest on one such catastrophe at Grantham but the coroner, although attributing the death to ether, exonerated the medical practitioner and regarded the method as legitimate. It was surprising that there were not more deaths but perhaps some were concealed from the public. Mr Lucas of Liverpool used ether to operate on a Newfoundland dog within a few weeks of its human application. Robinson published the first text book on anaesthesia early in 1847 but he is now forgotten despite the part he played. He deserves credit as the first to advocate the use of oxygen to counteract adverse effects of ether.[70]

The news of Liston's operation reached Scotland very quickly although, rather surprisingly, word of the Dumfries operation did not immediately spread. On the receptive mind of Simpson the discovery made an immediate impact. It has always been said that, from the start of his medical career, he had been searching for a means of relieving pain in surgical operations. Some surgeons, trained as they were to perform heroic procedures with almost incredible speed, may have

been strangely insensitive to the terrors of their patients operated upon in the conscious state but there were many as
humane as Simpson who must have longed for the new discovery.

Simpson, like other contemporaries, had been attracted by
the work of Anton Mesmer (1734-1814). This Austrian doctor
evolved a system of therapy based on his own undoubted
success achieved by what now would be termed medical hyp-
nosis. His cures by suggestion he attributed to the transmission
from doctor to patient of a vaguely defined force or 'animal
magnetism'. Suggestion was strengthened by an elaborate
ritual and by the use of magnetic appliances of all shapes and
sizes. Mesmer was not a charlatan, in the early period of his
career at least, but had a sufficient background of medical
training and experience to choose the right patient for this
psychiatric treatment. Unfortunately his system was such that
it was all too readily taken up by the quack. When Mesmer
died in 1818 there were many who believed in his methods
and indeed used them with intelligence. The practice of
mesmerism was relatively late in reaching England but found
a powerful exponent in John Elliotson (1791-1868) a London
physician of great wisdom and ability. James Esdaile (1808-
1859), an Edinburgh surgeon who practised in India for many
years, achieved remarkable success in hypnotising patients
so that they tolerated operations without pain. When Esdaile
returned to Scotland he found his fellow countrymen rather
more resistant to hypnotism than were his Indian patients!
Esdaile and James Braid of Manchester published convincing
reports on the value of the method in surgery. Simpson, either
because of his enthusiasm for a new idea or because of a particular interest in investigating any means of relieving pain
at operations, studied mesmerism thoroughly. He soon found
that he himself had exceptional hypnotic powers but he was
astute enough to appreciate that only certain patients would
respond and that only some diseases could be relieved by
suggestion. An early hope that mesmerism might permit of
painless surgery was soon dismissed and in time he realised
that the cult had far outstripped its bounds and that it had
fallen into the hands of unscrupulous practitioners who elevated it into a pseudo-science of electro-biology. As in his

subsequent exposures of the dangers and false claims of homoeopathy, Simpson in this investigation showed his unfailing common sense. He had a sympathetic understanding of the extraordinary credulity of the human race but he knew too well that such an ill-founded doctrine would inevitably multiply the quacks, qualified and unqualified. That mesmerism was very much discussed by the surgeons of this time is indicated by the remark attributed to Liston when he completed his historic case under ether, 'this Yankee dodge beats mesmerism hollow!'[71]

Simpson knew a great deal about the drugs used to relieve pain prior to the development of general anaesthetics and delved deeply into the classical writings. Apart from this and his interest in mesmerism there is nothing, however, to suggest that before 1846 he had performed experiments clinically or on animals in attempts to produce anaesthesia. When the news of Liston's operation reached Edinburgh, Simpson was probably quicker than most to appreciate the significance of the discovery. There is evidence that he went to London immediately to get direct information from Liston and that he brought back the necessary apparatus:[72]

When I saw Mr Liston in London, during the following Christmas holidays, he expressed to me the opinion that the new anaesthetic would be of special use to him—who was so swift an operator—as he thought, like Bigelow, it could only be used for a brief time. I went back, however, from this London visit to Edinburgh bent on testing its applicability to midwifery. . . .

Although Simpson wrote the preceding paragraph in 1870 it indicates strongly that as soon as he knew of the success of ether as an anaesthetic for surgical operations, he realised that it might also be used to relieve the pains of labour.

It is likely that Simpson told his friends all he had learned from his visit to London. Professor James Miller has been credited as the first to do an operation in Edinburgh under ether. He heard of the new discovery direct from Liston in a letter dated December 23rd. He read this to his class:[73]

Rejoice! Mesmerism, and its professors have met with a heavy blow and great discouragement. An American dentist has used ether (inhalation of it) to destroy sensation in his operations.

. . . Yesterday I amputated a thigh and removed, by evulsion, both sides of the great toe-nail without the patients being aware of what was doing, so far as regards pain . . . Shall I desire Squire: a most capital and ingenious chemist, to send you a tool for the purpose? It is only the bottom of Nooth's apparatus, with a sort of funnel above, with bits of sponge, and, at the other hole a flexible tube. Rejoice!

Simpson may have persuaded Miller to use ether as they lived near each other in Queen Street and despite the trouble over Miller's election they were again on friendly terms. Other surgeons in the Infirmary certainly used ether in the first two weeks of January 1847 and, even if they had no direct information, they all could have read the flood of reports in the London journals.

As might have been expected Syme was exceedingly cautious about this innovation. He was shown late in December 1846 a letter from Dr Boott to Professor Alison in which the use of ether was described. He later maintained that he was the first to employ it publicly in the Infirmary. In March 1847, when others had widely accepted ether anaesthesia for most operations, Thomas Cunningham, a student, wrote to his brother in describing how he had just seen Syme do two amputations and he noted that Syme: [74]

did not give ether—he has been averse to it ever since it was made known. The great reason was that he failed in the majority of his cases in producing insensibility and this arose from loss of patience. He now says he thinks it will not do, at least for capital operations.

This letter and other evidence suggest that Syme was certainly one of the first to make tentative trials with ether but that he was not carried along on the tide of enthusiasm which prevailed. In February he had expressed himself very cautiously and remarked that he 'did not attach much importance to extinction of pain during operations'. He stated unequivocally that 'good surgery consisted in carrying out more important objects than removing temporary pain and as far as his experience had hitherto gone he was not much impressed in favour of ethereal inhalation'. By March, as Cunningham records in his letter, Syme temporarily abandoned the use of ether in his clinic. By August he was, however, more or less converted to its use for he found if he used Simpson's technique he got better results. About this time he published six consecutive operations in which he had used ether with success but he was 'far from desiring to sanction its indiscriminate employment'. In September he was rather aggrieved when Simpson, in one of his articles, quoted his earlier remark on the negligible importance of pain in operations. He replied in the next issue of the journal with some dignity and with a statement which summarises his surgical philosophy: [75]

> I have been misrepresented as utterly regardless of the pain suffered by patients. Having consistently endeavoured to lessen the sufferings inflicted through the practice of surgery by diminishing the frequency of operations and simplifying their performance, I trust that any notice of a charge so unexpected, beyond an indignant denial, will be deemed superfluous.

Syme, despite his antagonism to Simpson, eventually became enthusiastic about general anaesthesia, particularly with chloroform, and was regarded as an authority on its use. As late as 1864, however, he did the horrific operation of removal of the tongue for cancer without anaesthesia, justifying this torture 'since the patient, instead of lying horizontally, might thus be seated in a chair, so as to let the blood run out of his mouth . . .'. But with such reservations he made full use of general anaesthesia and he recognised in it a great surgical advance.

Being an obstetrician it was not surprising that Simpson immediately applied anaesthesia in difficult labour. On January 19th, 1847 he gave ether to a woman who required a complicated delivery because of her deformed pelvis. Although the infant died the mother did well and had no pain during the operation. On the same day Simpson received the letter of his appointment as Queen's Physician in Scotland. Next day he wrote to his brother: [76]

> Flattery from the Queen is perhaps not common flattery but I am far less interested in it than in having delivered a woman this week without any pain while inhaling sulphuric ether. I can thing of naught else.

A preliminary report was published in February in the *Monthly Journal of Medical Science* and this was augmented in *Notes on the Inhalation of Sulphuric Ether in the Practice of Midwifery* in the March journal. The article was printed in pamphlet form and widely circulated. Not only did Simpson report on ether anaesthesia for labour requiring forceps or operative intervention but he also referred to several instances of its use in natural labour. While to use ether for operative midwifery was a natural extension of the rapidly accumulating experience in ordinary surgical operations, to use it for natural labour, merely to relieve the expected and accepted travail, was something quite novel. This was to bring down on Simpson's head the wrath of a large section of medical and lay opinion. Simpson at once allayed the fears of those who affirmed that if labour pains were controlled then uterine contractions would cease; after all it was known that on occasion regular uterine contractions could continue during natural sleep. He admitted that there was much to be learnt about the effect of ether on the mechanism of child birth but was soon convinced that it did no harm to child or mother, that by the relief of severe pain shock was diminished and that the method was as justifiable for operative midwifery as for other operative surgery. He came straight to the more difficult point, to answer those critics who so deplored his suggestion that the pain of normal labour should be relieved. Unlike some of his contemporaries he had no illusions concerning the intensity of pain which was often suffered in natural birth. He quoted Professor Naegele's description of the pangs of labour. 'They convulse the whole frame . . . the patient quivers and trembles all over. . . . Her impatience rises to its maximum with loud crying and wailing and frequently expressions which, even with sensible, high principled women border close on insanity.' He concluded: [77]

> Will we ever be 'justified' in using the vapour of ether to assuage the pains of natural labour? Now, if experience betimes goes fully to prove to us the safety with which ether, under proper precautions and management, be employed in the course of parturition, then looking at the facts of the case, and considering the actual amount of pain usually endured. . . . I believe the question will have to be changed in its character. For instead of determining in relation to it whether we shall be 'justified' in using this agent . . . it will become, on the other

86

hand, necessary to determine whether on any grounds, moral or medical, a professional man could deem himself 'justified' in withholding and *not* using any such safe means (as we presuppose this to be), provided he had the power by it of assuaging the pangs and anguish of the last stage of natural labour. . . .

He knew well that by writing this he would be involved in a long struggle against custom and prejudice. The struggle was to reach a peak after he introduced chloroform and perhaps he had little conception of the bitterness of the opposition which would develop. His self-appointed mission to convince his fellow practitioners that they should alleviate pain in normal child birth is the strongest evidence of his humanitarian feelings. Any fear that his campaign would damage his career, as well it might have done, was dismissed in his genuine desire to relieve human suffering.

In the compact community of Edinburgh the introduction of ether anaesthesia immediately became an exciting topic not only to the doctors but to the lay public. On February 17th there was a discussion at the Medico-Chirurgical Society. Syme gave his cautious opinions and many others got up and described their experiences. Some emphasised the risks such as convulsions, lung complications and explosions. On the whole there was wide acceptance for the use of ether, even in obstetric practice. The discussion was resumed on March 3rd with Syme giving an even less favourable report than before but there was enthusiastic advocacy from many others. Simpson described how he had used ether to control the severe pain of biliary colic. He reported too how he had observed its successful use in operations on horses. He was delighted at the rapidity with which the profession had accepted the new discovery. Professor Christison ascribed this to improved communications between doctors but Syme thought that they were all far too ready to adopt new ideas and were behaving very rashly.

The *Monthly Journal of Medical Science* provided frequent leaders on the progress of 'etherisation' and, although advocating caution, supported Simpson even in his application of the method in normal labour. The inflammable nature of ether was a cause for much alarm and Mr Young, a cutler, deserves recognition in the pages of medical history for he submitted himself to full anaesthesia and at all stages of his induction had a naked light applied to his mouth to prove that there was no danger of an explosion or of damage to his lungs! In these early months of 1847 many of the doctors tried out ether on themselves with considerable abandon and, surprisingly, no fatality!

Most of the clinicians like Syme based their opinions on their own experience of relatively few cases or were swayed by vague theories. Simpson adopted a scientific approach to the problems of anaesthesia. There was one other worker in the field who had this scientific approach and this was John Snow (1813-1858) of London, who attempted to make anaesthesia safer by measuring the optimum dosage of the vapour and developing accurate devices to deliver such doses. Simpson had three main objects in his researches in 1847. Firstly he wanted to prove, contrary to the opinion of many others, that ether anaesthesia made operations safer. Secondly he wanted to confirm that in obstetrics the anaesthetic was not harmful to mother or child. Thirdly he wanted to find a substance which was more effective and more manageable than ether.[78]

He set about proving the first point in a very simple way. Having evaluated as far as possible the mortality rates for major amputations in the main British and French hospitals prior to 1846, he then wrote to all the larger hospitals in Great Britain and asked for the mortality rates of amputations done under ether. He went to great trouble over this survey and asked for a special form to be filled in by each hospital. These returns are all preserved and in themselves are a fascinating record of this aspect of surgery in British hospitals at the time. Before ether was used Simpson calculated that the overall mortality of major amputations was 38 per cent for primary or immediate operations and 24 per cent for secondary or delayed operations. From his returns of 302 cases he calculated that with ether the mortality rate for primary amputations was 32 per cent and for secondary amputations 20 per cent. His contention that his figures proved that ether made amputation safer would not stand criticism from a modern statistician but at least he justified the statement, contested by many, that ether did not make surgery more dangerous. More important, in this survey he demonstrated the value of statistical analysis of large numbers of cases from a large number of sources. This was an important advance in the use of statistical studies in medicine.[79]

Simpson recorded his investigations in a series of three articles on 'Etherisation in Surgery' in the *Monthly Journal of Medical Science*. In the first article he attacked those who based their objections to anything new on 'mere opinions and prejudgements'. He retold at great length how Jenner had encountered futile arguments and theological obsessions when he tried to establish the value of vaccination but how when his work was accepted it had reduced the death rate from smallpox dramatically. He anticipated a similar struggle to establish the value of anaesthesia and insisted that only by the elucidation of accurate and well sustained facts could any such new discovery be established. He went on to stress the need to relieve pain in surgical operations and in child birth and exploded the fallacy that pain was a 'healthy indication'. The second article was a long dissertation on the importance of applying accurate statistical studies in the study of medicine and he showed himself well acquainted with the use of statistics in government and other fields. The third part was devoted to his comparison of amputation cases with and without ether. This part was, in fact, published two or three months after he had introduced chloroform.

Throughout 1847 Simpson used ether widely in obstetric work and by the end of the year had amassed a great volume of evidence in its favour. His advocacy of its use for the normal case was still greatly criticised and powerful opposition came, in particular, from some of the leading London obstetricians. Tyler-Smith, for example, came out strongly against Simpson but most of his arguments were ill-founded and he concentrated on obscure and irrelevant moral issues.

All the time Simpson was looking for something better than ether and those who have tended to regard his discovery of chloroform as a lucky chance forget that his trials with this substance were the culmination of prolonged experiments with many other volatile fluids. These experiments were crude and they could hardly be termed scientific. There are no records of animal experiments in this period but Simpson adopted the simple, if reckless, expedient of inhaling different drugs himself or observing their effects on his colleagues, his students or his patients. It is not too far fetched to suggest that in subjecting himself to all these experiments with gases and vapours, which were often exceedingly toxic, that he brought on much of his subsequent ill-health and accelerated his death. When in due course Simpson hit on chloroform in this rather haphazard research there were many, like Dr Ashwell, who deplored these reckless clinical trials and Simpson's habit of demonstrating his experiments at dinner parties and public meetings. He wrote to Dr Ashwell in March, 1848: [80]

> I have been laid up for the last twenty hours in bed, ill, and quite undone for the time, from breathing and inhaling some vapours I was experimenting upon last night, with a view of obtaining other therapeutic agents to be used by inhalation; and I write in bed. A few hours ago I received the *Lancet*. Your strange paper in it has done me the world of good. I have seen the time when such a scurrilous attack as yours would have irritated me. Nowadays such things produce the very reverse, so that I fancy I am getting quite hardened. . . .

To his family and friends these experiments must have remained a source of great anxiety. His butler found him on one occasion lying unconscious and is credited with the comment 'He'll kill himsel' yet wi' thae experiments: an' he's a big fule, for they'll never find anything better nor chlory'.[81]

The story of Simpson's discovery of the anaesthetic properties of chloroform has been described in colourful and dramatic detail and embellished over the years. Chloroform was known as a relatively pure preparation before 1847 and had a place in general therapeutics and Simpson made no claim to have established its formula or its preparation. It was more readily available in the impure form of chloric ether and before November 1847 Furnell, while studying pharmacology as a student, had inhaled this mixture and recommended it as an anaesthetic to the London surgeon Holmes Coote. Holmes Coote persuaded Lawrence to use it at St Bartholomew's Hospital but the trial was abortive and was not published in any detail.[82]

To Simpson chloroform was just one more volatile substance to which he was prepared to give a trial. He was the kind of person who if he met an expert on any subject always picked his brains. He very likely consulted with any chemist he might encounter about anything which might prove to have anaesthetic properties. In October 1847 he met Dr David Waldie then on a visit to Scotland from Liverpool. Waldie suggested that chloroform might meet Simpson's requirements and he offered to send a pure sample for trial. This he was unable to fulfil as about this date his laboratory was burned down and he lost all his equipment. From this episode arose an argument about priority which has continued until this day, for Simpson was accused of having failed to award to Waldie the credit due to him for the original suggestion to use chloroform.[83]

David Waldie (1813-1889) was born at Linlithgow, a few miles from Simpson's birthplace. He qualified as a doctor in Edinburgh in 1831 and so was likely to have known Simpson in his student days. In 1839 he gave up medical practice to become a chemist in the Liverpool Apothecaries Hall. He became interested in the preparation of chloroform when Dr Formby, a Liverpool doctor, sent in a prescription for chloric ether. As a chemist he was one of the few in England in 1847 who knew how to prepare pure chloroform; as a qualified doctor he was well equipped to discuss the therapeutic properties of the drug.

Shortly after Simpson first used chloroform he wrote to Waldie, 'I am sure you will be delighted to see part of the good results of our hasty conversation' and he enclosed a reprint of his first paper on the subject. In subsequent articles Simpson usually, but not always, recorded in a footnote that Waldie had 'named' chloroform as a likely agent. Waldie was of course extremely interested in Simpson's practical application of chloroform and on November 29th he read a paper to the Liverpool Literary and Philosophical Society on 'Chloroform: the new agent for producing insensibility to pain by inhalation'. In this he recalled his meeting with Simpson, 'chloric ether was mentioned. . . . I recommended him to try it, promising to prepare some after my return to Liverpool.' There was no amplification of this statement and Waldie at this time seemed content to accord to Simpson all the credit for the discovery. There is evidence that Waldie did some experiments on himself with ether and perhaps with chloroform but the date of these trials is uncertain and he did not report them at the time.

There was a meeting at the Liverpool Medical Institution on November 25th, 1847 when Dr Parke read a paper condemning the use of both ether and chloroform; Waldie was present and took part in the discussion but unfortunately there is no record of what he said. On December 28th Simpson and Waldie both attended a further meeting in Liverpool as the guests of Dr Petrie (who was related to Simpson by marriage). Simpson was received with acclamation and he gave a short account of chloroform after the main business of the meeting was concluded. There is every reason to believe that Simpson and Waldie were on good terms and, in fact, they continued to correspond in later years.

In 1852 Waldie went out to Calcutta where he practised with great success as a commercial chemist and for a while his small share in the development of chloroform was forgotten. He had, however, a brother George who was a chemist in Linlithgow and it was he, encouraged by David's former business associates in Liverpool, Clay and Abraham (of a well known pharmaceutical firm), who re-opened the whole argument. George Waldie published a pamphlet in 1870 in which he reprinted his brother's paper on the subject and made a strong plea for a greater recognition of his share in the discovery. There was an addendum written by David Waldie in which he recalled the events of 1847: [83]

> When news came I was pleased at my recommendation but was also mortified that from those unfortunate circumstances I had not been able to do something in carrying it out. I had inhaled nitrous oxide gas and ether vapour before—if I had been in a position to prepare chloroform I should at once discovered its properties on my own person. . . .

He now expressed regret that his suggestion to Simpson was mentioned only in a footnote, describing this as a 'parsimony of acknowledgement'. At the same time he admitted 'some of my friends have over-rated my share'. He did feel, however, that he deserved as much recognition in the discovery of chloroform as Simpson himself had accorded to Jackson for his part in the discovery of ether as an anaesthetic agent. David Waldie was a modest man and it is doubtful if he would have pressed his claims further had he not been harried by his brother. George Waldie emphasised that but for David's unusual combination of chemical and medical knowledge of chloroform, which was unique in 1847, Simpson would never have tried the drug.

All that David Waldie wanted was that Simpson should have admitted that in their conversation chloroform was 'recommended' and not just 'named'. Time and again this kind of quarrel over a priority revolved around a single word! Not until 1870 did David Waldie see himself rather hard-used and he wrote to his friend Abraham: [83]

> I was never satisfied with the recognition my share in the matter got, because I could never admit that the acknowledgement made by Dr Simpson was at all adequate. He did as little as he could possibly do and the statement was not a fair one.

When George Waldie's pamphlet came out it was noted in the medical press with sympathy but perhaps a statement in the *Lancet*, in an anonymous article on the 'History of Anaesthetic Discovery', should have closed the question: [84]

> Shall we take away the credit? It was Simpson who was looking for a new agent, it was Simpson's enquiry which lead Mr Waldie to think and suggest; it was Simpson who experimented with chloroform to prove it as an anaesthetic: and, lastly, it was Simpson who accepted the responsibility of the first introduction.

Family support and local patriotism were not in vain because in due course Waldie's work was commemorated by memorial tablets in Linlithgow and in Calcutta. A later Liverpool proposal to record his achievements suitably has not, however, come to fruition!

As things turned out it was not Waldie who supplied Simpson with a sample of pure chloroform but someone in Edinburgh. This may have been a chemist Thomas Smith of the firm of T. and A. Smith but Simpson suggests that the original sample came from Duncan and Flockart who in due course held almost the monopoly of the supply.

There is another version of the source of the historic sample of chloroform. Matthews Duncan was present when chloroform was first tried and in 1875 he wrote a letter to Robert Christison. In this he described how he had gone with Simpson to the laboratory of Dr Gregory, Professor of Chemistry, and had collected a variety of substances with 'respirable vapours'. Duncan experimented with these himself and: [85]

> took particular notice of chloroform as the best, and likely to be most useful, judging from its effects on myself. . . . In the evening I brought these bottles to Dr Simpson: and, supper being finished I drew his attention to the chloroform.

This is the only written evidence of the possibility, suggested quite strongly by some, that Duncan made himself unconscious with chloroform *before* Simpson had an opportunity to try it. On such evidence there are scarcely grounds for giving Duncan any more credit than is due to him for his participation in the historic events of the evening of November 4th. Some discrepancies in all these accounts are readily explained because the participants recalled the details many years after the event. In the autumn and winter of 1847 there were numerous meetings at Queen Street where, usually after dinner, the company conducted their somewhat dangerous experiments. On most of these occasions Dr Matthews Duncan and Dr George Keith were present but other participants may have been David Skae, Thomas Keith and possibly Professors Miller and Christison. Duncan and George Keith were, at the time, assistants to Simpson and it is reasonably certain that on the night of November 4th they, with their chief, inhaled chloroform. An account by Simpson in a letter to Dr Glover is probably as accurate as any and this indicates that some chloroform which a local chemist had supplied was tried out quite by chance: [86]

> In searching for another object among some loose paper after coming home very late one night my hand chanced to fall upon it and I poured some of the fluid into tumblers before my assistants Dr Keith and Dr Duncan and myself. Before sitting down to supper we all inhaled the fluid and were all 'under the mahogany' in a trice to my wife's consternation and alarm.

There are more elaborate versions but these are probably second-hand and some of the details may belong to the numerous other trials which were conducted about this time. Professor Miller, who was a near neighbour, apparently knew what was going on and was accustomed to call at Simpson's house in the morning to see if anyone had come to harm! He gave a more detailed story in which he described Simpson's immediate recognition, when he regained consciousness, that here was something stronger and better than ether. He recorded that Simpson woke up first but Duncan remained snoring under the table and Keith was in a state of high excitement and kicking violently. Mrs Simpson and three other relatives who were in the house at the time are said to have witnessed the startling scene and if so were not likely to forget it. The three experimenters soon pulled themselves together and had no compunction, it is said, in trying out chloroform on Miss Petrie, Mrs Simpson's niece, who obliged by falling into a deep sleep crying 'I'm an angel! Oh I'm an angel!'[87]

Simpson's reactions were immediate. Having used up all of the original bottle he at once induced the chemists of the firm of Duncan and Flockhart to manufacture more. Five days later he used chloroform on a midwifery case. Almost simultaneously his surgical colleagues, Duncan and Miller, were persuaded to use it for three surgical operations and Simpson gave the anaesthetics.

The discovery was announced to the Medico-Chirurgical Society on November 10th with Professor Alison in the Chair before a crowded meeting. On this notable occasion Simpson read a paper 'Historical researches regarding the superinduction of insensibility to pain in surgical operations: and announcement of a New Anaesthetic Agent'. He outlined the events which led to his trial of chloroform and stressed the advantages which he thought to be held by chloroform over ether. The small dosage required, the rapidity of action, the absence of irritating or exciting effects, the pleasant smell, the relative cheapness and ready portability of chloroform were enumerated. Finally he commented on the simplicity of its administration, advocating no complicated apparatus but that it should be poured out of the bottle into a hollow sponge or a handkerchief held in a cone over the patient's face. Already he could report its successful use in dental extractions as well as in midwifery. When he had read his paper Simpson

suggested that a committee should be appointed to test the
new drug. The meeting then became somewhat of an orgy: [88]
   The Society then adjourned when a very singular scene took
   place. Dr Simpson having stated that any gentleman who felt
   inclined might try the effects of chloroform on his own person,
   Mr Young, cutler, at once presented himself—after a few in-
   spirations complete insensibility was produced . . . several other
   gentlemen followed in succession. In one (Mr Hunter) some
   excitement was produced. He stood up and on being held made
   some resistance. He afterwards declared that the effect produced
   was similar to that occasioned by the nitrous oxide gas. Whilst
   the bustle attendant on this case was in progress, the handkerchief seemed to have circulated among the members, who
   applied it to their faces, and were unexpectedly surprised by
   the effects produced upon them: so that when we looked round,
   we saw more than one gentleman insensible and several others
   in various stages of apparent intoxication. They all, however,
   rapidly recovered . . . a few stated their sensations to have been
   so delightful that they should have no objection to their
   repetition.

The impact made by the first use of ether in Great Britain
was nothing to that produced by Simpson's announcement of
chloroform anaesthesia. The news travelled south with great
rapidity. On November 20th Simpson published a preliminary report in the *Lancet*. Within a few weeks he himself had
used chloroform for more than 50 cases of labour. Most of
the surgeons in Edinburgh at once discarded ether and even
Syme was quickly converted to the use of chloroform. The
committee, formed at Simpson's request, soon reported that
ether should be discarded. They did a series of experiments
on themselves and on willing students. Animal experiments
were conducted intensively with rather an odd selection of
subjects including 'a lively leech', 'a vigorous frog', 'a pigeon
and a dog'. With this report and the experience of his colleagues, recounted at the medical societies, Simpson's claims
were accepted almost unanimously in Edinburgh. Before the
end of the year the editor of the *Monthly Journal of Medical
Science* wrote that 'Ether seems already abandoned'.
   The publicity was tremendous and the lay public joined
in the excitement, alternating between fears of danger or
abuse and thanksgivings for the relief it offered. It became the

fashionable topic of conversation and Simpson's name was so closely associated with its discovery that he was hailed as a saviour of mankind and, by many, as the discoverer of anaesthesia. Allusions to the use of chloroform abound in the memoirs, biographies and novels of the period. Typical is a letter written by Lady Stanley of Alderley in Cheshire to her daughter-in-law in London in February 1848:[89]

> I do not like chloroform for teeth, I have heard of several cases where the experiment has been a very disagreeable one for the bystanders, and Alice's preserving a sort of consciousness throughout and being alive enough to *talk* rather makes me believe more than I had done in the account we read of some Edinburgh *experiences* where the young lady calls her dear Charles to come to her arms—and elsewhere I have heard that it is very desirable every body should have a friend with them and one who *may* hear anything that *may* come out during these trances. I think it is a *cowardly* thing to use it for tooth drawing only, and dangerous perhaps for nervous people. I think you certainly should not allow Blanche to try it. It is a very curious discovery and doubtless there will be a great improvement both in the preparation of the chloroform and the manner of applying it. I think the most extraordinary part of the business in this partial consciousness and Uncle confirmed it by an instance he knew of amputation, where a man talked of the operation all the time, like one looking on, yet felt no pain.
>
> Emma Mainwaring was delivered yesterday *without* chlo: and had the best and shortest labour she ever knew. She has been dissuaded from trying it—had she done so how they would have given all the credit of her good time to that.

Lady Stanley was well informed and up to the minute for she had ordered pamphlets on chloroform from the bookseller. She showed a fine degree of scepticism about it all and some of her comments were more intelligent than those of Simpson's medical critics. It does seem in England, as Simpson often said, that they were not very clever about the dosage! Emma Mainwaring too had gone into the question very thoroughly and had originally intended 'to be delivered without knowing it'. She had heard Dr Locock of London express approbation of chloroform 'as a boon not to be rejected' and medical men in Chester had encouraged her to have it. We remain in ignorance of why she changed her mind but at least this allowed Lady Stanley to utter the inspired statement at the end of her letter.

In Edinburgh the operating theatres were large and doctors and students often brought along their friends to witness operations. Even Dr Chalmers, the eminent divine, 'a presbytery in himself', witnessed an operation under chloroform. Nationally and internationally Simpson's name was enhanced and his discovery elevated him to a pinnacle of fame from which he was never to be dislodged. In London his advocacy of chloroform was seized upon with enthusiasm by the majority and those who opposed his ideas held objections not so much to chloroform as to the general conception of anaesthesia, particularly if given to relieve the pains of labour. Prominent amongst such critics was Dr Gream who brought forward ill-founded arguments that mother or child could be rendered idiotic, that the natural mechanism of labour would be impeded and worst of all that chloroform would 'excite improper sexual feelings and expressions in women'. He knew of 'several cases in which women under the influence of chloroform had used obscene and disgusting language. This latter fact alone he considered sufficient to prevent the use of chloroform in English women.' As Gream had just published a thoroughly unpleasant account of his treatment of sterility in women, some correspondents thought that his delicate feelings were misplaced.[90]

Simpson had all his answers ready for the critics, he had covered the ground thoroughly when he fought to establish the use of ether in childbirth. He had no difficulty in squashing the critics on technical aspects because of his own wealth of practical experience and the rapidly increasing corroboration of his colleagues. He soon had to turn his attention to another type of criticism which came from the moralists and the theologians. The intensity of this quarrel is difficult to appreciate today, but in the opposition to the Darwinian theory we can find a parallel illustrating the ferocity with which anything challenging Victorian ethics or religious beliefs was fought.

Simpson as the first to advocate the relief of pain in normal childbirth was attacked from the pulpit and in the press. He was inundated with abusive letters from cranks, from clergy-men and from colleagues. Some of the clergy, however, were on his side and amongst them was Dr Chalmers who thought that the 'small theologians' who took such an uncompromising and unmerciful view of the subject should be ignored. The opposition was powerful, however, and Simpson knew he must meet it. He produced many pamphlets and in these he was not afraid to attack the theologians on their own ground.

Those who were against the relief of pain in childbirth based their beliefs on the writings in *Genesis* and particularly on verse 16 of the third chapter, 'Unto the woman he said, I will greatly multiply thy sorrow and thy conception: in sorrow shalt thou bring forth children. . . .' They interpreted the word 'sorrow' as pain and would not permit that this 'primeval curse' should be removed from the human race. Simpson studied the Hebrew texts and concluded that the original word should be translated as labour or toil rather than pain. Whether his interpretation of early Hebrew words is right or wrong remains uncertain. He was on safer ground when he compared the objections against anaesthesia to those, equally ill-founded, brought against vaccination. He argued that if the physician was justified in using a drug like mor-phine to relieve pain, what moral difference was there in relieving pain by the inhalation of chloroform or ether? He slipped a little when he quoted from *Genesis* 'And the Lord God caused a deep sleep to fall upon Adam: and he slept: and he took one of his ribs, and closed up the flesh instead thereof.' This he cited as the first description of a surgical operation and he quoted from various authorities to suggest that the Creator induced sleep to relieve pain. Dr Ashwell, one of his critics, took this rather seriously and was quick to point out that Adam could not have experienced pain anyway as the operation was performed during the state of man's innocence and before the introduction of pain into the world![91]

Some of Simpson's arguments may have failed to convince the theologian but by his persistent writing and his persuasive character it can be said without question that he won the battle almost on his own. In the end it was the strong humani-tarian argument which prevailed and it was the patient who came to demand anaesthesia. Much has been made of the fact that when Queen Victoria had her ninth child, the Duke of Albany, she accepted the relief of chloroform. While this certainly must have had great influence in fashionable circles and indeed put the seal on Simpson's success in the eyes of the world, this notable event did not take place until 1853. By this time most of the doubters had been quelled.[92]

If we look at these events in retrospect, with all the advantages of modern knowledge of anaesthetic substances, we can see some things very clearly. First of all there is no question that chloroform is easier to administer than ether in that the initial stages of induction are accomplished without the irritation and excitement induced by ether. Secondly it is easier to maintain a patient under deep anaesthesia with chloroform than with ether. Chloroform has now, in fact, been almost totally discarded as an anaesthetic partly because there are many new anaesthetic agents which, with modern techniques, are more effective. The main reason for discarding chloroform, however, is that in the occasional instance it induces sudden death and that this may occur after a very small dosage. Further there is evidence of dangerous side-effects on the liver, particularly after heavy dosage.

If Simpson had one great weakness as far as chloroform was concerned it lay in his absolute refusal to admit that it could ever be dangerous. He is not the first, however, to have become obsessed with an attitude of infallibility about a technique or a therapy of his own invention. The enthusiast often builds up a barrier against criticism of his ideas and this may be only human in his intense desire to establish what he genuinely believes is right. Simpson never forgot an early experience when having planned to give chloroform for the first time for a surgical operation, he arrived late to find that the surgeon had started without him and that the patient had died after the initial incision. To him, therefore, an anaesthetic death could often be explained by the operation. In his refusal to admit that chloroform could kill, he became involved in bitter arguments which, we must accept, revealed a blind and obstinate streak in his understanding. Some clinicians soon became aware that chloroform was potentially dangerous and it was not long before fatalities were announced in the medical press. In Newcastle, early in 1848, a young girl, Hannah Greener, died while being given chloroform for a trivial operation. Much has been made of this case as Simpson took it upon himself to suggest that she died from asphyxia when her medical attendant tried to force some brandy and water down her throat. Simpson may have been right about this as inhalation of fluid by an unconscious patient can cause sudden death. His critics said, however, that he was falling over backwards to deny the possibility that the death was due to chloroform. There were many cases like this but undoubtedly Simpson felt that if any doubt was cast on the safety of chloroform, in which he believed implicitly, his whole campaign to establish the use of general anaesthetic would be ruined.[93]

Despite his masterly exposition of statistical methods, when he surveyed the amputation series Simpson deceived himself, and was held to deceive others, when there was much discussion about the relative incidence of deaths from chloroform in Scotland and England. For a while he denied that any death had happened in Scotland. Eventually he had to admit that a few had occurred but that there had been far more in England. He forgot to make allowances for the much larger population in England and that inevitably far more operations were done there. John Snow attacked him very justifiably on this point and in doing so demolished the arguments that only in Edinburgh did they know how to give the drug safely or that the London chemists manufactured an impure brand.[94]

While the arguments never really subsided it is fair to say that for some 50 years chloroform was the most popular general anaesthetic. It is not without significance that when a new operating theatre in a London hospital was planned as late as 1890, the anaesthetic room was labelled the chloroform room. When the statue to Simpson in Princes Street was erected the engraving on the plinth read 'Discoverer of Anaesthesia'. (This was corrected in 1947.) Simpson himself never pretended that he did more than develop general anaesthesia by applying it to obstetrics and by introducing chloroform which had so many advantages over ether. He was always ready to acknowledge the work of the American pioneers such as Morton and when in 1869 Dr Bigelow accused him of trying to claim all the credit for the establishment of general anaesthesia this was a mean and unjustified attack. Simpson's contribution was immense and apart from his purely technical achievements he must have recognition for his part in defeating the prejudices against this major advance of medical science in the century.[95]

In 1850 Simpson became ill with an abcess originating from a septic finger, the occupational hazard of surgeons of the time and, not so infrequently, of fatal consequence. An operation was necessary and Simpson wanted to call in Professor Miller. But Mrs Simpson had other ideas and she persuaded her husband to consult Syme as the most skilled surgeon available. That Simpson agreed to this indicates that he respected Syme's ability and superiority as a surgeon. That Syme was willing to help in such a crisis suggests that he could rise above the quarrels which had so often darkened their relationship. Presumably Simpson was given chloroform and it would be interesting to know who was the anaesthetist, doubtless he was well briefed by the patient! The operation was successful although Simpson's recovery was slow and demanded a long convalescence.

CHAPTER 7

Controversies and Current Affairs
(1750-1860)

I N 1848 Syme became President of the Medico-Chirurgical
Society and in 1850 President of the College of Surgeons.
In the same year Simpson was elected President of the
College of Physicians. It was not unusual at this time, and
for many years afterwards, for a physician-accoucheur to hold
this appointment. During Simpson's tenure of office there was
a complete revision of the laws of the College and no doubt
he played a considerable part in these negotiations. In 1853
he, in turn, became President of the Medico-Chirurgical
Society and meanwhile continued to hold office as President
of the Obstetrical Society. Both men were therefore in positions to exert a great influence on all medical affairs.

The middle years of the century were marked by rapid
advances in medical science but these were to some extent
confused, or even overshadowed, by the introduction of many
new doctrines contrary to orthodox teaching. At a time when
registration was non-existent and when almost anyone could
practise medicine, the dangers of such cults and fashions
were well recognised. Three particular groups of unorthodox
practitioners sprang up at this time; the mesmerists, the
hydrotherapists and the homoeopathists. It was homoeopathy
which had the greatest impact and which led to the greatest
arguments.

The German Samuel Hahnemann (1755-1843) propounded
a doctrine with which was associated a novel form of therapy.
In his *Organon*, first published in 1810, he laid down certain
laws. The first law was 'like cures like' or *similar similibus
curantur*; that to cure a disease it was necessary to use a
remedy which produced in a healthy person symptoms similar
to those of the disease itself. In diagnosis, therefore, there was

little or no place for established principles of anatomy, physiology or pathology. The second law was that the medicine selected should be given in infinitesimal dosage, for if standard dosage was given the substances selected would aggravate the disease process. Hahnemann advocated the utmost dilutions possible and defined effective 'potencies' or 'attenuations' prepared by elaborate techniques. For example, 2 drops of a chosen material might be diluted with 98 drops of alcohol; the dilution was increased by adding 1 drop of the first tincture to another 99 drops of alcohol; the process was repeated several times until a tincture was obtained in which the allegedly potent substance was present in a proportion which was expressed by a millionth or even a decillionth. The effectiveness of the dose was said to be enhanced by a precise ritual of shaking. The patient was given the medicine to swallow or in some instances merely smelt it! Alternatively 'globules' were prepared by incorporating minute quantities of the chosen material in starch or sugar. The third principle was that only one pure substance should be given at a time; this was technically difficult to ensure, if not impossible.

Hahnemann convinced many doctors (and some remain convinced today) that his theory and practice were legitimate. He cured a proportion of his patients and the reasons for his partial success are readily apparent. Firstly, in the majority of human ailments there is recovery because of natural resistance. Secondly, at a time when patients were so often over-dosed with medicines the substitution of a régime of rest, fresh air and simple diet (part of Hahnemann's prescribed routine) was often dramatically successful. Thirdly, as with mesmerism, the factor of suggestion could be curative in some diseases. It is fair to see in the introduction of homoeopathy an important counter to the abuse of drugs, known to the homoeopaths as allopathic medicine. This abuse was in fact well recognised by many contemporary physicians, such as Robert Christison, Professor of Materia Medica in Edinburg, who campaigned against it in a more orthodox fashion than Hahnemann.

To most physicians homoeopathy presented a considerable challenge and when the cult extended to become quasi-religious it seemed to many that it had gone too far. The early disciples of Hahnemann ascribed to him a supernatural power. At one school of homoeopathy students were admitted to the select circle with the words 'In the name of Hahnemann, discoverer of Homoeopathy, from whom I have received the mission and the power and with the assistance of my coadjutors, the disciples of that messenger from Heaven, I now declare you fit to exercise the new art...'. Hahnemann taught that disease depended on a perversion of spiritual power and that the infinitesimal dose released a spiritual effect which was not to be obtained from standard dosage.

It must be recalled that the nineteenth-century doctor was powerless in his ability to cure or even control many diseases for which we now have specific remedies. He was well aware of the dangers of many popular drugs; mercury, for example, was used to such excess that the hospitals were often crowded with those suffering from the terrible effects of mercury poisoning rather than from their original diseases. In an age of rapid change many doctors were all too ready to seize on anything new, for even the doctors shared in the general gullibility of the human race. But an acceptance of homoeopathy denied almost all established medical teaching and any thinking clinician had to make a choice. It was not surprising that to the leaders of the profession everywhere it was soon very clear that an attempt should be made to establish the reliability or otherwise of Hahnemann's teaching. To the over-confident or bigoted there was no problem and the practice was categorically denounced, just as some denounced Harvey when he propounded his theory on the circulation of the blood, Jenner when he introduced vaccination, or, in later years, Lister when he tried to establish his antiseptic doctrine. To the small group of the gullible, which exists in every age, a sweeping new theory with a mystical flavour was readily acceptable. To the thoughtful there was an urge to give any new idea a fair hearing or even a trial. All such doctors existed in every country and while stressing the world-wide impact of homoeopathy it is relevant here to describe the repercussions only in Edinburgh and the part played by Syme and Simpson in the controversy.

The teaching of Hahnemann filtered to England and Scotland in the late thirties but for a while received only sporadic and superficial attention. At first it was received with the same scepticism and even ridicule which had greeted mesmerism and it was not seen as a serious rival to current philosophy or technique. Most believed that when the novelty wore off the system would be forgotten. The quackery of James Graham with his Temple of Health, his exploitation of sexual deviation and excitement and his theatrical use of electrical apparatus had not survived for long. 'Perkins Tractors', a relatively mild piece of mumbo-jumbo by which the hysteric or the readily hypnotised might be cured by the manipulation of two metal rods, had come to England from America but were soon forgotten.[96]

In 1845 a leader in the *Medical Times* expressed a fairly typical attitude in England towards homoeopathy: [97]

> And what is homoeopathy? What is the new system of cure found out six thousand years after Adam, which is deemed worthy of the royal patronage. . . . It is the old thing over again. It is a science that has something new, but that something is not true; that has something true but that something is not new. . . .

In 1851 the Provincial Medical Association did not take homoeopathy very seriously, although it deplored the support it derived from an idle and bored aristocracy and from a small group of Church of England clergy. But there were many individuals who before this date saw dangers in the wholesale support of homoeopathy. They recognised how readily it could be exploited by the unscrupulous: they appreciated too, that a deep responsibility lay on medical teachers if the new doctrine was encouraged. There were, of course, vested interests and not surprisingly the pharmacists saw in the new therapy a threat to their enormous profits. By the late forties it was becoming a serious matter for any surgeon or physician of repute to be known as having consulted over a case with a confirmed homoeopathist. The journals of the period are full of letters with such accusations and with hot denials from those so blamed.

In Edinburgh there was an explosion of some magnitude. The trigger was the appointment, largely owing to Simpson, of William Henderson as Professor of Pathology. Henderson had beds in the Infirmary and taught clinical medicine as well as pathology. In 1844 he professed homoeopathy. The implications were obvious to the Faculty and at once it had to consider the effects of Henderson's teaching on students. He published in 1845 *An Enquiry into the Homoeopathic Practice of Medicine* which was one of very many such pamphlets, but because it emanated from a professor engaged in active teaching in a school of the importance of Edinburgh it was singled out for attack. The *Lancet* was particularly scathing and deplored that a professor of pathology should maintain that a disease could be cured by ignoring the underlying pathology: 'every intelligent student cannot but regard the chair of pathology, and the lectures delivered from it, with a feeling very much approaching contempt'. The *Edinburgh Journal of Medical Science* wrote of Henderson, 'his talent misapplied, professional dignity lowered and a popular delusion left as hopelessly in the mind as ever'. The attacks on Henderson were to persist for years and London was ready to censure the University severely for allowing such an anomalous situation to continue. Henderson, in fact, retained his chair until he retired in 1869 but in 1844, the Faculty, headed by Syme as Dean, remonstrated with him and he had to give up his clinical teaching in the Infirmary. The Faculty had no direct control over the Chair of Pathology as this was under the patronage of the Town Council.[98]

Many of Henderson's colleagues, including Syme and Simpson, were greatly embarrassed for over the years they had consulted with him professionally and so laid themselves open to the charge of supporting homoeopathy. At this time the Edinburgh Medical School was in any case subjected to much abuse and criticism and there had been a falling off in the number of students. Everyone was extremely sensitive about all this and Henderson's activities demanded positive action.

In 1851 the College of Surgeons, under Syme's presidency, denounced the homoeopathists, as did the College of Physicians under Simpson. The London colleges, although so critical of Edinburgh, did not take this drastic step. The licensing bodies felt powerless because they could not prevent a candidate from obtaining an orthodox degree or diploma and then immediately practising homoeopathy.

It fell to the influential Medico-Chirurgical Society to take further action and at a meeting in December 1851 Syme proposed 'that the public profession of Homoeopathy shall be held to disqualify for being admitted or remaining a Member of the Medico-Chirurgical Society of Edinburgh'. Syme thought it quite unnecessary to discuss the principles of homoeopathy, he assumed that all the members, like him, had formed adverse opinions. He devoted much of his speech to defending himself against charges that he had collaborated with Henderson in the past. He recalled how he had been greatly exercised when Henderson became a convert and how he, as Dean of the Faculty, had insisted on Henderson's resignation from the Infirmary.

Simpson seconded the motion. Having quickly cleared *his* name from any association with the homoeopathists he embarked on a lengthy attack on Hahnemann's doctrines. It was clear that he had devoted a lot of time to the study of the subject. He drew a vivid parallel between the homoeopathists and the Mormons but his main attack was on the law of the infinitesimal dose. He appealed to 'the standard of common sense' in quoting the 'strangest contradictions and wild absurdities' of the therapeutic doctrine and he ridiculed the techniques used by homoeopathists by his elaborate and quite bewildering mathematical calculations. He just refused to believe that drugs in millionths, billionths or decillionths had any effect. Most of all Simpson stressed how the preparation of these minute doses was open to fraud and he cited examples where either it had been proved that there was no active ingredient at all in the preparations or a homoeopathist had played for safety and given the accepted allopathic dose. Henderson was let off lightly but Simpson did recount how a friend had sent him a handsome case of homoeopathic drugs. He had given this to one of his children and in play the drugs had been mixed up. One day Henderson saw the case and took it away and used it in his practice, with great success!

For once Simpson and Syme were united and their influence was such that the Society accepted the motion unanimously. The result was positive as far as Edinburgh was concerned and orthodox medicine had triumphed![99]

For Syme the matter was closed, his opinion had been

formed and no further argument was required. For Simpson it was quite otherwise, if he embarked on a controversy he followed it to the bitter end. He saw it as his duty to continue public opposition to something he regarded as false and fraudulent. Some influential person had to clear the air and Simpson with his ability at probing into the history of a subject, his cogent powers of reasoning and his strong personality was just the man. He marshalled his facts in great detail and in 1853 published the first of repeated editions of *Homoeopathy. Its tenets and tendencies, theoretical, theological and therapeutical.* This is a lengthy volume and is not particularly well constructed but, by its demolition of Hahnemann's theories, its critical analysis of the results of treatment in the established homoeopathic hospitals and its exposure of the swindles perpetrated by unscrupulous practitioners, it proved a very effective document. From his study of mesmerism Simpson was well aware of the credulity of mankind and how there were 'no absurdities too groundless to find supporters. Whoever determines to deceive the world may be sure of finding people to be deceived. . . .' He was very much aware of the place of the 'vis medicatrix naturae' in any régime and he granted that Hahnemann had laid down excellent dietetic and hygienic rules for the management of disease. He gave credit to Hahnemann for his part in forcing doctors to look afresh at drug therapy and to recognise the abuse of dangerous drugs. The work is not without humour for in criticising the technique of giving homoeopathic drugs by 'olfaction' Simpson relates how, in settling the account with her practitioner, a lady 'subjected to the process of olfaction passed the fee before his nose and then—replaced it in her pocket'. Simpson's message was quite clear:

> . . . homoeopathy stands perhaps unequalled in extravagance with any system of delusion than has, in any former times of ignorance and darkness, formed an object of human credulity and belief.[100]

The work involved in preparing this volume must have been enormous. It swamped the author in a vast correspondence, sometimes favourable to him but often critical or abusive. He gained wide support from the medical profession and many regarded his exposure of homoeopathy as one of his most important contributions to medical science. Some of the clergy were against him, the Reverend Everest of Wickwar in particular, who preached in support of the homoeopathists and who headed a petition in favour of a candidate for the Edinburgh M.D., who was rejected because of his homoeopathic beliefs. Pamphlets were exchanged in great numbers and Henderson replied to Simpson's publications with great energy, admitting however that he did not believe in *all* that Hahnemann had taught. It was largely owing to Simpson's campaign that homoeopathy, although never completely discarded, was reduced to minor significance and continued to attract only a few doctors.

It was inevitable that the two acknowledged leaders of the profession in Edinburgh became involved in other medical affairs of national importance. From 1830 attempts had been made to introduce a bill in Parliament for the better regulation of medical education and practice. The relationship between the universities and the various corporations was confused, the standards of education throughout the country were variable, there was no medical register and the public were quite unprotected from the unqualified practitioner and the quack. In 1843 a bill was presented to the House of Commons by Sir James Graham, but it met with great opposition from the general practitioners, incited to action by Thomas Wakley. This bill, had it been passed, would have ensured domination by the Royal Colleges by the establishment of a council largely composed of Crown-appointed professors and nominees of the Colleges.

Syme with his intense interest in medical education played a considerable part in the movement towards medical reform. This he did although his relations with influential London colleagues were scarcely such as to favour co-operation. He went out of his way to insult Dr Paris, the President of the London College of Physicians, by accusing him of having used an ex officio position on a committee to award himself the Swiney Prize for a work on medical jurisprudence. Syme used this incident to illustrate incompetence and corruption in the London colleges. There may have been some truth in his accusations but he had to apologise. Syme did not help his image with the College of Surgeons either, for he affirmed that he had been reluctant to accept the Fellowship granted to him in 1843. Despite such tactlessness he exerted considerable influence, even in London. His tactics were to write to those in high places and to make sure that his memorials were well publicised. In 1849 he addressed the Lord Advocate of Scotland, complaining of the restrictions imposed on Scottish graduates who wanted to practise in England. This was one of the many anomalies which demanded correction but it was unfortunate that Syme in making his plea decried the quality of the teaching and the qualifications of the English schools and attributed perfection to the Scottish schools. When he affirmed that the teaching staffs of the London schools were drawn entirely from their own men, it was not surprising that the London journals hastened to remind him that he and his predecessor Liston had been appointed to London from outside. In this document, however, there was much wisdom, for Syme proposed that the government should appoint a board to be termed the Medical Council with powers to regulate the education required for the general practitioner, to control the licensing of all practitioners and to establish a register of qualified doctors. Some were alarmed at the prospect of the Board of Health choosing such a council and deplored that Syme offered no representative principle by which the doctors would elect their own members.

In 1853 he sent a somewhat similar memorial to Lord Palmerston. Although this too was criticised for its partisan attitudes it contained the principles which were largely accepted when in 1858 the bill for the Reform of Medical Education was finally passed. Syme was in due course appointed to the new Medical Council as the representative of the Universities of Edinburgh and Aberdeen. He retained his seat on the Council until 1868, proving an active and constructive member even though at times his outspoken criticisms of others exceeding reasonable limits.

Simpson exerted an influence on the reform movement in a more subtle way. For many years he corresponded privately and intimately with those such as Lord Elcho, Sir Charles Hastings, Mr Cowper, Dr Markham, Dr Forbes and Dr

Storrar who were deeply involved in medico-political affairs. It is significant that when Headlam's bill was passed in the House it was Simpson who was able to secure an important amendment by a last minute dash up to London.[101]

It was appropriate that the new bill was announced to the profession in Edinburgh at the annual meeting of the British Medical Association. By 1858 this had become the important mouthpiece of the profession. After it was founded in 1832 by Charles Hastings (1794-1866), in Worcester, as the Provincial Medical Association it was subjected to much criticism, but in time its activities and influence had expanded. Scottish branches were late in being formed and at first there were few members North of the Tweed. Simpson was one of the first Scottish members, having joined as early as 1844, and he had attended some of the English annual meetings. Syme had joined in 1853 but when at the annual meeting in Oxford, a surgeon, Hester, commented adversely on the litigation then in progress between Syme and Lizars, Syme took this as a personal insult and resigned. Simpson wrote an angry letter to the Association in which he gave Syme his full support and he at least threatened resignation. When the Association held its annual meeting in 1858, for the first time in Scotland, Syme had not rejoined it but Simpson was to play a prominent part.

Sir Charles Hastings arrived a few days before the meeting and stayed at Simpson's house. There must have been much talk and excitement about the chances of the Bill being passed. Some 150 members attended the meeting, including many like Hastings, returning to the scenes of their student days. Professor Alison, now aged and ailing, was the President. He gave rather a dull address, but he was received with acclamation and respect. While the progress of the reform bill dominated much of the interest there was time for the discussion of a variety of topics. Simpson gave the address on obstetrics while Professor Miller gave the address on surgery. This perhaps kept Syme rather out of the lime-light but many went to see him perform an excision of the tongue and the English visitors were 'much pleased with the cool manner he performed a very bloody if not difficult operation'. In addition Syme conducted a clinic which Christison reported as 'masterly'. The climax of the meeting came on the Friday afternoon when an urgent despatch was handed to Simpson. The contents were at once shown to Hastings who announced, amidst loud cheers, the final passage of the medical reform bill.[102]

The annual dinner that evening was a great occasion. The aged Alison was not able to preside and his place was taken by Professor Christison. There was justifiable gratification at the part played by the Association, particularly through Hastings and Simpson, in bringing the reform movement to fruition. Hastings made a moving speech when his health was proposed. Simpson proposed the health of Vose of Liverpool, the President-elect for the next year. There was a very long toast list, even longer than usual for these affairs. They drank the health of even the King of Sardinia, which was just explicable as the Sardinians had been staunch allies in the Crimean War. The company showed a remarkable capacity for withstanding endless speeches, aided by the lavish flow of bumpers of champagne. The proceedings were enlivened by musical interludes with Christison, Bennet, Peddie and Maclagan providing a professorial glee party. Christison records how an unknown Liverpudlian doctor: [103]

> a little em-port-é came up to him at the end of the festivities and said 'I see now how your countrymen thrive wherever they go. You are a devilish deal cleverer than we. Why? Because besides all else you have given us a treat such as we never got before. Why, I tell you what it is doctor, we might visit every town in all England and we would not get a chairman and three of his townsmen to give us such a feast of music'.

The party might have gone on far into the night had not Christison announced that the Provost of Edinburgh had left and might return with the police to enforce the laws of Scotland which demanded that such gatherings should disperse at 11.0 pm!

Most of the reports of the meetings were enthusiastic and highly appreciative of Edinburgh's hospitality. The reporter of the *Medical Times*, however, was a little sour about it all and complained that the dinner was poor and the wine indifferent. In all this jollification Simpson played the part of the genial host and captivated the English visitors. Syme was less prominent but some of those from London may still have regarded him with a degree of suspicion.

In 1854 the Crimean War broke out. Even before Russel, the correspondent of *The Times*, exposed the gross deficiencies of the army medical organisation the doctors in Edinburgh were roused to excitement and many volunteered to serve abroad. This was the first major war to involve Britain since Waterloo. To the younger men the chance of active service offered novelty and adventure with the possibility of acquiring in a short time a practical experience denied to them at home. An intense wave of patriotism swept the whole country and reached a peak when the Russians destroyed the Turkish fleet at anchor at Sinope in November 1853. There were many ways of joining the army. A permanent commission had little appeal because of the slow promotion, the long periods of service abroad and the poor pay and status of the junior officer. It was, however, remarkably easy to obtain a temporary attachment for the campaign through influence. Some doctors sailed for the East armed only with a letter of introduction to the Colonel of a regiment.

An early volunteer was Richard Mackenzie (1821–1854), an assistant surgeon in the Infirmary, trained by Syme and already rivalling his master. Mackenzie had a particular motive for he hoped by surgical experience in the field he would enhance his chances of succeeding the aged Sir George Ballingall in the Chair of Military Surgery. He left for the war in June 1854 and joined the 79th Highland Regiment at Varna. The army suffered heavily from cholera before it embarked for the invasion of the Crimea and there was little surgery to be done. Mackenzie wrote to Simpson at this time and expressed the hope that there would be an abundant supply of chloroform. He landed to take part in the battle of the Alma and in a few hours of hectic surgery did 32 'capital' operations—including two amputations at the hip joint. Next day the regiment asked permission to give their surgeon three cheers in recognition of his work. Two days later he was dead, struck down by cholera. Mackenzie's death had important repercussions because it created a vacancy at the Infirmary which was filled in 1856 by Joseph Lister who had come to Edinburgh three years previously to work under Syme.

Mackenzie was older than most of those who volunteered for service just before the outbreak of the war. That there were many young volunteers is shown by the fact that of the resident staff of the Royal Infirmary in 1854 Lister alone remained behind while his colleagues Heron Watson, Alexander Struthers, John Beddoe, John Kirk, George Pringle and David Christison all went out to the Crimea. Lister at the time was a Quaker and it would have been against his principles to serve with the army in any capacity. As things turned out his apparent evasion of this unofficial draft was very much to the benefit of humanity!

To both Syme and Simpson the problems of the medical organisation of the army must have been of great interest. Simpson seems to have been more actively involved. His advice was sought at every stage and he engaged in much correspondence with Lord Palmerston, Lord Panmure and Sidney Herbert. It was suggested that the catastrophic situation should be met by the despatch of surgeons and physicians in civilian units to be attached to the army. A group of doctors, mostly from London, including such notable men as Holmes Coote and Spencer Wells, went out and ran civil hospitals first at Smyrna and later at Renkioi in the Dardanelles. It was announced that Simpson had carte blanche from Lord Palmerston to establish a second unit but the plan was not executed. He and Syme used their influence to select suitable individuals to go out as junior regimental officers. A letter written late in 1854 by Simpson, with instructions to the young doctors Greig, Johnston and Alexander Struthers, illustrates the patronage of such appointments. It also shows how Simpson used every means to collect information about the things in which he was interested: [104]

> I do not know if this will reach you in time but I hope it will.
> Dr Storrar will have also told you that Lord Blantyre has written about the money and I suppose you have already received £50. . . .
> Be so kind and remember that Lord Blantyre's conditions simply are:
> 1st. that you write me now and again how matters go with *you* and with the sick.

2nd. That if his brother—the Honble Mr Stuart an officer in the Rifles is wounded or ill—you 'will be kind enough to pay him special attention.'

3rdly. Lord B's sister—Lady Seafield has a brother-in-law an officer in the 47th (Mr Grant) for whom he and his sister would fain have equal privilege.

Further he wishes the chloroform taken out. They have not nearly enough there. And I hope you will be able to show them how to use it properly.

Please let me ask of you as a personal favour to make any incidental enquiries you can about the existence of leprosy (Elephantasis Graecorum) in Turkey or the Crimea. Have they anywhere Hospitals for lepers—and which symptoms does the disease principally exhibit? I have heard that one of the Greek islands is used as a Lazar or Leper House.

Dr Storrar has £10 over. If you can lay it out on Hennan's Mediterranean (a model military medical work) or Pringle's Campaigns or Larrey's works—please be so kind as to expend it on these or other books as a present from me. And if you take notes of the *diseases* as well as the wounds etc.—I do not see why one of you or all of you, conjointly, or separately should not write an excellent essay (medico-chirurgical) on the campaign.

I feel sure that three more energetic and more able young medical officers will not be found in the East.

One point more. Pray take care of your health and do not unnecessarily overwork or expose yourselves. If you meet with any difficulty that Lord Blantyre, Mr Syme or I can remove— write at once to me.

May God bless and prosper you and believe me that no one feels more deeply interested in your prosperity, success and well being than

Yours ever faithfully,
J. Y. Simpson.

Simpson was of course particularly anxious that the army doctors should be well supplied with chloroform and should know how to use it. For a campaign of this type chloroform had great advantages over ether as it was less inflammable and as only small quantities were required. In September 1854 John Hall (1795–1866), Director of the Army Medical Services in the Crimea, issued a directive about chloroform and this with a general memorandum to his staff was re-

printed for all to read in the *Illustrated London News* of
September 23rd 1854: [105]

> Dr Hall takes this opportunity of cautioning medical officers
> against the use of chloroform in the severe shock of gunshot
> wounds, as he thinks few will survive where it is used. But
> as public opinion, founded perhaps on mistaken philanthropy,
> he knows is against him, he can only caution medical officers
> and entreat they will narrowly watch its effects: for however
> barbarous it may appear, the smart of the knife is a powerful
> stimulant: and it is much better to hear a man bawl lustily
> than to see him sink silently into the grave.

Hall became the scape-goat for much of the Crimean
fiasco but many of the accusations against him were unjust.
At the end of the war Miss Nightingale was particularly
harsh in her criticism of him and made sure that he did not
succeed Andrew Smith as Director-General of the Army
Medical Services. He was of course to some extent justified
in his recommendations about chloroform and was reflecting
an opinion held quite strongly by many surgeons at home.
Charles Clay, a notable pioneer in ovariotomy, wrote as late
as 1863 that he was averse to using chloroform and stated
'if it could be accomplished I should infinitely prefer to
operate without it, as the patient would bring to bear on
her case a nerve and determination to meet so great a trial,
which would assist beyond all value the after treatment. . . .'

Hall's directive was regarded by many people as ill-judged
and inhumane and a prohibition against the use of chloroform. It was Syme who reacted immediately and in a terse
letter to *The Times* of October 12th, after quoting Hall's
guidance, he wrote: [106]

> If this statement were limited to its influence to the particular
> occasion, it might not require any notice: but as such doctrine
> if intensively promulgated without contradiction, would have
> a far wider range of effect, it seems requisite to state, as a
> result of long and ample experience in opposition to what Dr
> Hall *thinks* on the subject, that chloroform does not increase
> the dangers of operations performed during a state of exhaus-
> tion, however extreme: that pain instead of being a 'powerful
> stimulant' most injuriously exhausts the nervous energy of a
> weak patient; and that, therefore, so far as the safety of the
> operation may be in question, chloroform proves useful directly

in proportion to the severity of the injury or disease and the degree of exhaustion or shock.

In due course chloroform was used extensively and successfully by the military surgeons both in the front line and in the base hospitals. When at first it was in short supply Simpson arranged for many medical officers to take out a personal stock of the anaesthetic. Dr Dowson of the Guards, for example, was supplied with a whole case of chloroform and perhaps justifiably Simpson was rather annoyed when he learned that having taken this to the Crimea not only did Dowson not use it but he did not pay for it! When the war ended there were numerous reports emphasising how essential chloroform was in military surgery and testifying to its safety.

Simpson had first-hand information from the young men from Edinburgh for whom he had negotiated temporary attachments to the army. Amongst them was Alexander Struthers who went out to Scutari in November 1854 and worked all the winter in the desperate conditions of the base hospitals. He wrote many letters to his brother John Struthers as well as to Simpson. In some of these he criticised the work of Florence Nightingale and her nurses. He made amongst other observations reference to Miss Nightingale's religious beliefs and this came to the notice of those in authority in London. There were plenty of rumours about the behaviour of the nurses at Scutari and Miss Nightingale was suspected of sectarian intrigues. Mr Sidney Herbert felt it necessary to defend her and letters were exchanged with Simpson in an attempt to clear up the affair. Simpson defended his protégé and he wrote to Professor Bowman, who was intimately concerned in the nursing organisation: [107]

> . . . whoever stated that Dr Struthers spoke in his letter of Miss Nightingale as an Unitarian most *maliciously* misrepresented Dr Struther's letter. He talks of her as a 'good protestant', he speaks of some of the nurses she brought as 'invaluable' or 'Godsends' etc.
>
> I believed with you that Miss Nightingale and those that accompanied her went out as 'nurses' and nurses only; and nobody admired them and their mission *more* than myself. But Dr Struthers who is a man of the greatest probity and

honour—as well as of the highest professional talents states plenty of facts to shew that they have assumed, or *pretended* to assume, at least, the character of spies upon the medical men as well as nurses to the patients—noting down the time the patients are dressed etc. and (in one case of Miss Nightingale's) going to the Superintendent physician and making him send down an order for a patient to be dressed by his surgeon out of turn, instead of applying to the surgeon himself etc.

All this is so totally against proper co-operation—mutual respect—and the honour of the medical officers that it will inevitably lead—sooner or later—to bitter strife—unless it be at once stopped—and the ladies reduced to their true character of nurses and nurses only—Dr Struthers casually mentions about Miss Nightingale keeping a man lying on the operating table for 15 minutes *till* she could be found—as she wished to be present at all operations. In such a matter there is at least a great want of judgement on her part—and a want, I think, of proper discipline on the part of the medical officers. . . . In Dr Struthers' ward were three of Miss Sellon's sisters—but he was only allowed to speak to one of them. Only think of nurses in a ward when the physician was not to speak to. Could there be anything—or any mal arrangement *more* intensely ridiculous and absurd? I do believe that the sooner this and other matters are re-arranged, the better will it be for all parties—the patients, the nurses and the physicians.

Professor Christison was involved also and must have seen Struthers' letter for he wrote to Simpson: [108]
I presume the paragraph in Struthers' letter that has so much offended Mr Herbert is the following in P. 4 'She may be a lady but I don't think she has the modesty of anyone deserving to be called a woman'. This combined with the story of the operation at which she 'assisted', is more than enough to rouse the bitterest resentment of those who believe her to be an Angel or Heavenly-minded female. . . . If Struthers' letter get wind, the lady's relatives will never forgive him even if he is wrong, but, least of all, if he is right. And whatever the issue they will have influence and perseverance enough to effect his ruin. . . . *I* would say, it is not 'heavenly-minded Angels' that are wanted in Scutari,—nor tongue-tied Sisters with crosses and malignant looks neither,—but horny-handed nurses, strong, active and willing.

Christison advised Simpson to go to London to seek an

interview with Herbert to satisfy him that Struthers was a reliable and honest man. Perhaps rather foolishly Simpson sent Struthers' offending letter to the Minister of War and he received a cool reply defending Miss Nightingale's actions. Herbert denied that she had spied on the medical officers or criticised them in any way: [109]

. . . There is one other subject to which you have alluded i.e. Dr Struthers' statements that the Nurses are not allowed to speak to him in the discharge of their duties in the wards.

I know no one who is so free from the nonsense which is sometimes unfortunately apparent in some of the English Sisterhoods as Miss Nightingale—but I must say that any one who knows what young surgeons and medical students are as a Body must allow that too great caution cannot be exercised when young men and young women are thrown together amid such scenes in a male hospital.

As to Dr Struthers himself, I am afraid, . . . that he is hardly prepared for the kind of work in which he is now engaged. . . .

It is clear that Simpson shared the views held by many of the medical officers at Scutari. Some of these, from Dr Hall downwards, sent a flow of letters to London complaining of Miss Nightingale's autocratic behaviour, resenting her immense power and suspecting her of wielding undue influence by direct communication with the politicians in London. If any action was contemplated against Struthers it was too late for he died of a fever in January 1855, nursed tenderly in the terminal stage of his illness by Miss Nightingale herself. Simpson seems to have been much more aware than Syme of the lessons to be learned from the failures and fiascos of the war. He was particularly interested in the planning of the prefabricated hospital designed by the great engineer Isambard Brunel which was erected at Renkioi and administered by Edward Parkes (1819–1876). This hospital had features which Simpson had long advocated and he regarded the design as ideal for the prevention of hospital infection. Syme, rather surprisingly, despite his interest in amputations, in the management of wounds and all the other surgical problems which were discussed so freely at the time, made little or no public comment. He must have met many of his former students and assistants when they returned from the war but whatever he learnt from them he did not enlarge upon. Apart from his outburst against Hall's order about chloroform he intervened only in one other direction. When Ballingall resigned from the Chair of Military Surgery in 1855 Syme wrote to Lord Panmure advising that the Chair of Military Surgery should be abolished and suggesting that a new one should be established at a military centre such as Chatham where there was a close contact with the army. The proposal was accepted and in general it was a sensible one. There would have been, however, some merit in retaining the Chair in Edinburgh a little longer for although the war had ended there was still a large army of occupation, medical recruits were still urgently required and those sent out were often ill-equipped for their task. As the Professor of Military Surgery had beds in the Infirmary and did private practice Syme's motives may not have been entirely altruistic. Syme must have been interested in the work of Florence Nightingale and in the new impetus given to the organisation of nurses in civil hospitals. When Miss Nightingale after her return from the war undertook her intensive survey of the major hospitals in Britain she came to Edinburgh. It was Syme who received her and conducted her round the Infirmary and in later years she expressed her appreciation of his great courtesy and assistance.[110]

University affairs occupied the time and energy of both professors. They carried on clinical and systematic teaching with their original vigour and their classes were as crowded as ever. The election of new professors, as always, afforded scope for much rumour and intrigue and often the two men were in opposition. Edinburgh was much criticised concerning the power of the Town Council in many of these appointments and Simpson, a beneficiary of the system, defended its patronage in 1857. Syme exerted his influence by direct approach to the Secretary of State.

When Thomas Laycock (1812–1876) succeeded Alison as Professor of Physic in 1856 he was strongly supported by Simpson. Soon, however, Laycock suspected that Simpson was manoeuvring to relinquish the Chair of Obstetrics and to become a Professor of Clinical Medicine, in rivalry as a consultant physician. Edinburgh seemed fated to a kind of musical chairs! No sooner did a professorship become vacant than someone from another chair seemed to be ready to move in, or, there was a strong influence from some quarter to abolish the vacated chair. It may be charitable to suggest that some of these machinations represented genuine attempts to rationalise the teaching structure but one fears that behind it all there was jealousy which was largely tied up with a fear of losing a share of private practice. It was not only on the medical appointments that Simpson exerted his influence but he intervened in other faculties. His critics said he had inherited Thomson's title of the 'chair-maker'. When his friend Edward Forbes, Professor of Natural History, died in 1854, Simpson did his best to persuade the government to appoint Jean Louis Aggassiz (1807–1873) in his place. Aggassiz, one of the foremost biologists of the time, was then Professor of Zoology in Harvard and it was an imaginative stroke on Simpson's part to try and entice him back to Europe. Perhaps it was Edinburgh's loss that Simpson was not successful on this occasion.[111]

Simpson's involvement in all such elections came from his great prestige, nationally and internationally. The first thing anyone did when seeking any kind of appointment in Edinburgh was to write to him seeking his support. He may have enjoyed the power he exerted but it was in his nature to assist all who called on his services. Not surprisingly he incurred much bitter criticism and was often accused of sharp practices in these matters. At times his generosity may have outrun his political wisdom.

Every few years the opportunity recurred for the principal professors of the medical faculty to address the year's graduates. Syme was the Promotor in 1852 and having congratulated the new doctors he proceeded to give them stern advice. He insisted that in their early years after qualification they must work hard and eschew the pleasures of life, otherwise they could not hope to contribute to the advancement of medicine. He reminded them of the gullibility of the profession and the current tendency to adopt vague theories such as those of mesmerism and homoeopathy. He warned them that having accepted their degrees after orthodox studies if they adopted some obscure doctrine such as homoeopathy their duty was 'to strip off the doctor's gown'. While he cautioned them against making money by a sacrifice of their principles, he admitted it was easier 'to be virtuous in comfortable circumstances than under the pressure of want'. He continued 'I would earnestly warn you against the most fruitful source of debt and difficulty, which is an early marriage.' In short his message was that there was nothing ahead for the newly fledged doctor but concentration, hard work and a divorce from the pleasures of life.[112] (The critics said that he advised against marriage only because in a previous graduation address a colleague had spoken of this favourably!)

Simpson gave the annual address in 1855 and he ranged over a wider field. He foresaw that most of his audience would enter civil practice and discouraged them from going into the services. He criticised severely the meagre pay awarded to the military surgeons, a subject much under discussion at this time. He warned that in civil practice of any kind there would be a struggle to make ends meet and he quoted at length the early penury of great men like Astley Cooper and Benjamin Brodie. Like Syme he exhorted the graduates to work hard in their early professional career and affirmed that only in this way could they rise above mediocrity. In fervent terms he proclaimed the nobility of the medical profession, in his opinion ranking only second to the clerical profession which stood 'in unspeakable importance above the medical, and above all other professions, inasmuch as the interests of the soul are infinitely more momentous than the interests of the body'. He was reflecting contemporary feeling when he said that the easiest way to worldly fame and 'a corner in the peerage book' was for a man 'to destroy diligently and successfully, as a soldier, as many as possible of his fellow men'. He contrasted the awards to the famous generals with the meagre recognition of a doctor such as Jenner who had saved, rather than destroyed, so many lives. In these remarks he indicated the new sense of values infiltrating the Victorian Era. Simpson was particularly delighted to record the successful qualification of Dr Wong Fun, the first Chinese to graduate at a British University. He rejoiced that he and others of the many foreign graduates present would go back to their far countries and spread their knowledge of modern medicine. He ended on a high note of oratory: [113]

> We despatch you as Argonauts across the rough sea of life—not in search of a shadowy Golden Fleece,—but with a far higher and holier commission viz., to carry hence the rich blessings of medicine to all ends of the habitable globe, to give, as humble agents under a Higher Power, ease to the suffering, strength to the weak, health to the sick and sometimes life to the dying.

This was the kind of homily to which such audiences were well accustomed. The sincerity is without doubt and already Simpson was revealing an evangelistic and religious trait which was to become more prominent in his later years. Both Simpson and Syme had had their struggles in their early lives and both were at pains to warn the young of the trials ahead.

Despite all these preoccupations both men continued to practise their specialties with remarkable intensity and to publicise their ideas in a continuous stream of papers and lectures. In the two years of his presidency of the Medico-Chirurgical Society Syme contributed to one journal alone 45 lectures and cases of interest. After years of virulent criticism towards Syme the *Lancet* announced in 1854, that it would 'bury the hatchet' and, in praise of 'Syme's nobility in continuing to teach as his conscience demands, despite criticism . . .', inaugurated the publication of a long series of his clinical lectures. These covered the wide range of Syme's experience and he had no compunction in continuing his attacks on the methods of the English surgeons whenever there was the opportunity. When the lectures were completed the editor expressed himself delighted and said there was no one like Syme. Some of the things Syme wrote incurred censure, as for example when John Snow demolished the inaccurate statistics from which Syme, and Simpson, suggested that there were more chloroform deaths in England than in Scotland and that they did not know how to give chloroform in England. It was left to Joseph Lister to answer some of the other criticisms, particularly those of Syme's theories about club foot. Lister, in fact, was by this time preparing many of Syme's articles for publication and in every way was becoming his right hand man. It was not surprising that Syme's writings roused his opponents to wrath for he could be very personal in his case reports. In reference to a patient with a tumour of the mouth he wrote: [114]

> Lord —— applied to me on account of the excessive distress and haemorrhage caused by the disease—had spent two months in London under the care of Mr Bransby Cooper, Mr Travers and Mr Caesar Hawkins—all of whom, separately and collectively regarded his case as incurable and hopeless. He then applied to me—

Syme was not the only one who indulged in this open criticism of others, especially when they gave up a case as hopeless or made some error. But he did seem to overdo it! Despite this his reputation increased and he was achieving international fame particularly for his work on bone and joint diseases and on aneurysms and for his heroic surgery for advanced cancer of the jaw and tongue.

It was almost inevitable that there would be more litigation and perhaps it was because the laws of libel were different in Scotland than in England that it was an Edinburgh quarrel which brought about a major action. In 1849 Syme had published a small monograph *On stricture of the Urethra and Fistula in Perineo*. This was quite a brief account of 11 cases of obstinate stricture of the urethra which he had treated by a method of external excision which, in his opinion, was far better than by any other method. As this was a chronic condition which tended to recur despite any treatment he was perhaps a little hasty in stating 'of all the cases only one followed by unpleasant result'. The follow-up period was very short and he laid himself open to criticism when he recorded cures only one month after operation. The subject was a controversial one, Syme's beliefs were questioned by other authorities and the reviews were often unfavourable. The bickering between Syme and the London experts reached quite a high level of insult and arrogance and a climax was reached when Syme published a challenge. It was his contention that there was no such thing as an impermeable stricture, that is to say he believed that it was always possible for an expert to pass an instrument through the contracted channel of the urethra. Syme wrote to the *Lancet* in 1850: [115]

> I beg to express my readiness to receive into the Royal Infir-
> mary of Edinburgh any patients who may bring with them
> certificates, from a London Hospital, of labouring under
> impermeable stricture, I shall be happy to pay their expenses
> in coming and returning by steamboats which sail twice a
> week and would afford the most comfortable conveyance for
> invalids frequently disturbed with calls to make water.

The solicitude for the comfort of the miserable sufferers
is touching but it was not surprising that there was an uproar.
The *Medical Times* wrote that 'a surgeon of unsavoury
urethral notoriety assures the world that the London surgeons cannot pass a catheter properly'. John Gay, one of the
London surgeons most severely attacked by Syme, warned
anyone who thought of accepting the offer to go to Edinburgh: 'First make your will!' No one accepted the challenge
and soon attention was diverted to a major battle brewing
in Edinburgh. There were doubtless many who hoped that
at last Syme was to be the loser in a court action which
received much notice everywhere. The pursuer was none
other than the unfortunate John Lizars. He had lost his
professorship in the College and his appointment in the
Infirmary but he had struggled on as a rival to Syme in
private practice. His contributions to surgery had diminished
but he too was interested in stricture and published his book
on the subject in 1851. In this work he criticised Syme's
results and implied that his reports were inaccurate, particularly with regard to the incidence of serious complications
following his operation, the rate of recurrence and the
mortality. Lizars had already, in 1850, published letters in the
medical journals suggesting that Syme had concealed certain
cases in which his new operation was a failure. When Lizars'
book appeared Syme lost no time in launching an attack.
He wrote to the *Medical Times*, which had taken up the
cudgels on Lizars' behalf. The editor refused to publish the
letter in its entirety because he thought it was actionable
but Syme had it printed in the *Monthly Journal of Medical
Science*. He denied Lizars' accusations but the critical paragraph in the letter was as follows: [116]

You say a fierce paper war has arisen between the two Edinburgh professors Syme and Lizars; but you must or at least ought, to know that I have not addressed a single word upon the subject in question to the so-called 'Professor', regarding him *as being placed beyond the pale of professional respect and courtesy.*

Lizars considered this as a libel on his professional character and his position in society and the case was heard in July 1852. The counsel for the pursuer affirmed that a statement of this sort from one as influential as the Professor of Clinical Surgery in Edinburgh was bound to damage Lizars' reputation and he said that Syme knew very well he was incurring the risk of being accused of libel since the London editor had refused to publish his letter. He called witnesses, including Professor Miller and several general practitioners, who testified that the sentence could not be interpreted other than as injurious to Lizars. Counsel for the defence made much of the fact that everyone knew of the longstanding feud between Lizars and Syme and that accordingly Syme's statement merely repeated something which was already common property. He called as witnesses Christison and Simpson both of whom testified in favour of Syme. It was a little surprising to find Simpson appearing in Syme's interest but since Simpson's operation and illness they had been on rather less unfriendly terms than usual.

The jury pronounced in favour of the defendant. Reading the report of the trial in detail there is a strong hint that this was a miscarriage of justice and that Syme owed the verdict to his powerful position and influence: the defence excused Syme's statement on the grounds that Lizars had in his book made an unprovoked attack on Syme but the justification for this attack was never proved or disproved in court. Lizars was already a rather pathetic figure struggling to retain a place in surgical practice and the case well-nigh finished his career. The affair did not bring credit to either party or to Edinburgh. As usual the London journals took sides, the *Medical Times* against Syme, with whom it had other quarrels, the *Lancet* was against Lizars. Although Syme won the case many deplored 'the peculiar spirit in which he discusses the doctrines of others'. The *Medical Times* wrote of 'Syme's overweening conceit'.[117]

It might have been thought that the unpleasant publicity of this quarrel with Lizars would have restrained Syme from further strife. This was not so and as the years went on there were many more quarrelsome situations, some were petty but some concerned matters of principle. Syme did not always win as for example in the case of Glover v. Syme when he accused a police surgeon of issuing a certificate about a patient without having examined him properly. Syme fought this case in the firm belief that reform was urgently required with regard to the official procedures of taking medical evidence. He had to pay £250 in damages and heavy costs but most observers thought that the law had miscarried and they admired Syme's firm stand in the matter.[118]

There were countless quarrels in the correspondence columns of the medical press but it must be recognised that any surgeon or physician in the mid-nineteenth century who was not so involved could hardly be considered of any importance. When Spencer Wells became editor of the *Medical Times* he rather carelessly allowed the publication of a letter from an obscure practitioner who accused Syme of concealing the facts of the death of a private patient, a nobleman in Fife, following a fistula operation. Syme threatened litigation because in fact the account of the operation was quite false. He was of the opinion too that it was quite wrong to publish details of private patients. Spencer Wells, on the other hand, deplored the 'sanctity of private practice' and insisted that if anyone published the results of a particular operation he must include both hospital and private patients. As far as the accusations concerning mismanagement of the case were concerned Spencer Wells had to retract and an apology appeared in very small print.

After all his attacks on the London surgeons it seemed almost rash of Syme to set foot in the capital. In 1853, however, he addressed the London Medico-Chirurgical Society on the controversial subject of chronic stricture. Despite everything the London surgeons received him well, although a few were conspicuous by their absence. Even the *Medical Times* regarded the visit as the 'great event of the week' and wrote that there had been an 'amnesty proclaimed by the Imperial Autocrat of the Caledonian Capital'. In surgical circles at least the true worth and ability of Syme was now well recognised and his frequent vituperative outbursts were beginning to be taken less seriously.

From 1850 onwards Simpson with all his interests and diversions worked at his specialty with undiminishing energy. His private practice was time-consuming and involved him in long journeys up and down the country but he never wasted a minute, writing up his notes in uncomfortable railway carriages or in the periods of waiting for train or steamer. He continued his observations and experiments on anaesthesia, testing new drugs but was mainly concerned in amassing evidence of the superiority of chloroform. He became interested in the possibilities of local anaesthesia, particularly by the application of chloroform vapour or carbon dioxide. To the local societies he contributed countless case reports of obstetric and gynaecological problems. In the medical press he published many clinical lectures covering the whole of obstetric and gynaecological practice. He was friendly with Spencer Wells who as editor of the *Medical Times* commissioned a long series of articles on the diseases of women. There were wider interests developing on the problems of hospital infection, of wound healing and of the methods of controlling haemorrhage but Simpson's active entry into these controversial fields was not to come until after 1860.

The more Simpson wrote the more he was likely to be involved in discussion or argument. Many of his rather fixed views on chloroform were questioned by John Snow, the acknowledged London expert. A few diehards continued to attack the idea of giving anaesthetics for any reason. There was some truth in the charge that general anaesthesia had encouraged reckless and unnecessary operations. Professor Meigs of Philadelphia was a vociferous critic of the use of chloroform in natural birth and Simpson had to go over all the old ground in answer to his charges.

As a strong advocate of the use of the uterine sound and the speculum in the diagnosis of gynaecological conditions Simpson was the recipient of much abuse. 'Isaac Irons,' whose identity was uncertain, denounced such manipulations as an offence against all womankind. Lee was another such critic but he was rather swayed by the fact that the speculum was invented in France: [119]

> The speculum emanates from the syphilitic wards of the Hospitals at Paris and it would have been better for England had its use been confined to those institutions.

Dr Lee challenged Simpson on many of his theories and practices, particularly those relating to haemorrhage at childbirth from the abnormally situated placenta. Simpson's ideas on this subject were in fact somewhat shaky. He in turn attacked Lee on his elaborate anatomical studies of the nerve supply of the uterus, the validity of which is still in question.

The outcry which greeted any obstetrician or gynaecologist who advocated the use of instruments or techniques which might offend the delicate susceptibilities of English womanhood was something which impeded progress. This came from the gentlemen, not the ladies! Similar attitudes were shown towards the introduction of operations for the removal of the ovaries, such procedures were regarded by many as quite criminal. Simpson had more than his share of these attacks from prudish and perhaps hypocritical colleagues. In 1862 a book was published entitled *Stories of the Temple in Edinburgh*, printed in London and with the authorship concealed under the pseudonym 'An Acolyte'. It was suppressed at publication but a few copies were circulated. The foreword indicates its purpose: [120]

> This book . . . will be pronounced one which is on the side of virtue: yet we are compelled to the admission that we are sorry to have had the necessity put upon us of writing it. . . . It cannot be said to be of small importance to the virtue of a people that their wives, who are to be the mothers of their children, should be free from the reproach even that lesser shame of confidences in things which all nations have sealed with the signet of secrecy . . . the enactions of disease demand a certain sacrifice of feelings of delicacy, but the mere desire to become a mother can never authorise revelations *ex parte*, which must compromise the interests of a husband, and betray the deepest and dearest secrets of his heart.

Simpson, with his humane outlook, had devoted much energy to the problem of sterility. The first chapter is quite

an erudite and amusing survey of the history of the treatment
of infertility. The style is undoubtedly a caricature of that
employed by Simpson in the long and learned historical
introduction to most of his major papers. There are references to Edinburgh obstetricians such as Dr Thatcher, of
whom a jingle is quoted:[120]

>When a barren woman comes to me
>I give her bread pills and the devil take her
>But the never a guinea *I* take as a fee
>For I am a doctor, and not a baker.

Just in case the reader does not understand the allusion
there is a footnote to the word baker: 'a personal allusion to
some practitioner, we suspect'. The book is clearly seen as
an attack on Simpson. His busy consulting room is described
as the 'Temple of Fecunda':[120]

>There arose suddenly a great institution in the heart of the
>metropolis of Scotland. The fame of the mystagogue extra-
>ordinary . . . was heard of in foreign lands and honours
>rushed upon him so numerously that he might have been
>excused from doubting the reality of his divine mission . . .
>a secular confessional where matrimonial confidences are
>betrayed.

The remainder of the book provides a fascinating series of
case reports. Ladies from all ranks of society flock to the
oracle to be cured of sterility, from the young and elegant
English wife of the aged and drunken Highland laird to the
middle-aged thwarted spouse of an unfaithful Glasgow grocer.
More doggerel:[120]

>For Mrs Q's
>Has heard the news
>That in our metropolitan city
>Fecunda's art could make a barren
>Woman as fruitful as a warren.

>Whether the pills she got were wheaten
>We do not know: it was not written.
>Away she goes with her gilded box
>And surely a duty never could hoax.
>And nine months hence a pretty poupée
>Would pay her well for her honorarie.

Admitting the poor quality of the verses the text is, in fact, highly entertaining. But this is one of the most vicious attacks ever perpetrated on an individual even for an age in which professional abuse was commonplace. Simpson was slandered and denounced as a charlatan, as a money-grubber and, by ill-concealed innuendo, as a completely immoral person. It seems likely that he saw the book. If he did read it then he must have been deeply hurt. Although so much of his correspondence is intact no reference can be found about this slander, either in regard to its suppression or to its possible authorship. It may well remain an unsolved mystery but it is a memorial to the jealousies, the ill manners and sordidity of professional relationships in this period.

Although Simpson managed to keep out of the law courts he had his full share of trouble. There was a regrettable quarrel with Professor Miller which received much publicity and led to a weary correspondence. In March 1853 Simpson operated on the wife of a doctor and she died two days later. It was not unusual then for a surgeon to do an operation and if anything went wrong another consultant was called and the surgeon was not further involved. In this instance Professor Christison was summoned and he diagnosed a 'low peritonitis' as the cause of death. There were many rumours and then Professor Miller announced that the patient had died of haemorrhage and that Simpson had been negligent. Miller was not a vindictive man but he is said to have been offended that Simpson had asked Syme to operate on him in 1850. More likely Miller, as other surgeons, did not approve of Simpson extending his activities outside those of obstetrics. The quarrel became public property and most were on Simpson's side because Miller and his supporters quoted in evidence of a haemorrhage a statement from a 'common tradesman', an upholsterer, who cleaned the mattress of the deceased! Simpson was cleared of negligence and the husband of the unfortunate lady wrote to exonerate him completely.[121]

It may well be asked how these two men stood up to the perpetual strain of their busy lives. These were the years of maturity during which both had attained the positions they had so eagerly sought. In 1860 Syme was 61 and Simpson 49, the patterns of their lives were set but for another ten years they were to continue to contribute widely to medicine and their influence was to increase. It is convenient to pause here and to recount something of their domestic backgrounds and their interests outside medicine.

CHAPTER 8

Private Lives

I N the years during which Syme and Simpson rose to fame
progress in all branches of science was bewildering and
there was a social revolution. A great expansion of communications aided the exchange of ideas and travel at home
and abroad became more comfortable and more rapid.
Although spared the incessant demands of the telephone the
surgeon of this time could be summoned rapidly by tele-
graph when about 1855 this remarkably efficient mode of
urgent communication became established in Britain. The
penny post, inaugurated in 1840, greatly encouraged correspondence and was highly efficient. The growth of the rail-
ways although at first offering somewhat uncomfortable and
unsafe travel was by 1855 well developed. Before 1840 the
Edinburgh citizen who wanted to visit London was well
advised to go by sea from Leith, a journey taking about four
days and to avoid the tedious discomfort and slowness of the
posting coach. By 1845 it was possible to travel from Edinburgh to London by rail in less than two days but a night
had to be spent in York. By about 1855 the direct rail link
involved a journey of only 16 hours. All these changes were
linked with industrial expansion, increased foreign trade and
the exploitation of an Empire. The Great Exhibition of 1851
showed to the world just what Britain had achieved. Deeply
involved as they were in their medical interests Syme and
Simpson both must have been well aware of the surge of
events. To Syme changes were to be examined with caution
and perhaps were at times resented. To Simpson, to the end
of his days, changes brought excitement and were to be
exploited.

134

The domestic life and outside interests of Simpson are better known than those of Syme. While Simpson preserved most of his correspondence and his affairs were dutifully recorded by his family after his death, the personal papers of Syme were either destroyed or are undiscovered. The exuberant personality of Simpson was such that references to him abound in the writings of countless observers: the reticence of Syme was such that his private life and thoughts were known only to a select few.

The professional life of Syme revolved round his consulting room and the Infirmary. Paterson describes how he was an early riser and started the day with a visit to his garden. He then wrote his letters and breakfasted at 8 AM. He often walked from Millbank to his consulting room at Rutland Street. In the intervals of his consultations during the morning he read *The Times* in its entirety. The rest of the day was spent in the Infirmary operating or teaching. His work completed he returned to the oasis of his home and garden. His services were in demand all over Scotland and in the North of England and his ordered routine was interrupted by journeys which might take him far afield but having completed a consultation or done an operation he would return home as quickly as possible. Membership of the General Medical Council demanded frequent visits to London but these he accepted as a stern duty and the business completed he took the first train home. He was not often seen at medical gatherings such as the annual meeting of the British Medical Association and his somewhat parochial attitude on medical matters was perhaps extended to the broader aspects of life. He wrote in 1851: [122]

> I have long suspected and am now fully satisfied that neither Paris nor London possesses any hospital which affords so good a field for surgical observation as the Royal Infirmary of Edinburgh.

He did take regular holidays but was content with simple expeditions to the Highlands or to North Wales. He never went abroad after his early trip to the Continent although he had many contacts with foreign colleagues who visited him in Edinburgh. In 1863 he revisited Ireland and went to

Dublin. Despite some acrimonious affairs with his Irish colleagues in previous years he was well received and at short notice a dinner was arranged in his honour at which his health was drunk with lavish praise for his contribution to surgery. But in general he shunned public affairs and the oracle had to be consulted on his own ground in Edinburgh.

His domestic life revolved around Millbank where his chief joy was in his garden and greenhouses where he cultivated rare plants, fruit-trees and shrubs. Dr John Brown records 'matchless orchids and heaths and azaleas, bananas, and grapes and peaches'. He tells too the touching story of Syme's deathbed when knowing that one of his rare orchids would be in bloom he summoned his faithful gardener Paterson who brought the radiant flower to the sick-room; 'he gazed at it and bursting into a passion of tears, motioned it away as insufferable'.

It is only through the writings of the few intimates like Brown that we can penetrate to the true character of Syme, to find that he did not lack sentiment and that he felt for his fellow-men. From Brown too we learn of Syme's delight in the country; 'I went with Professor Syme to Peebles and had a delightful walk in the hills.'

His family life was private and those who knew him well described Millbank as the happiest of homes. The tragedy of the loss of first wife in 1840, almost certainly from puerperal fever, has been recorded. To the outside world he disguised his sorrow but, greatly exercised over the care of the two surviving children of this marriage, he married again. He found in Jemima Burn a happy choice for she was a kind and amiable person who entered into all his interests. The second Mrs Syme died in 1869, a year before her husband, and of her five children a son, James, survived.

Social life did not interest Syme greatly although in his practice he had a fair proportion of the noble and the famous. There were quiet dinner parties at Millbank with a few select friends or with his assistants and at times there were distinguished visitors. Thomas Carlyle came to Edinburgh in 1868 and Syme did a minor operation on him. Carlyle stayed at Millbank for two weeks and when he was convalescent there was a small dinner party. John Brown was present and he records that after dinner Syme more than held his own in conversation with the literary giant, as they sat on the low trellised verandah on the south side of the house watching the sunset over Blackford Hill.[123]

Through John Brown, Syme had contacts with the world of literature but there is no direct evidence that he read much outside medical subjects. Most of the notable Victorian surgeons or physicians, in their writings or recorded speeches, delight in literary allusions which give an indication of their tastes, but if Syme was at all scholarly or addicted to the popular classics of the age of this we can find no trace. It may well be that here, as in other matters, he was reticent and although well aware of all that went on in the world he formed his own tastes and judgements and remained aloof from public discussion and criticism.

There was one occasion at least when the entertainment at Millbank was lavish in the extreme. The British Association met in Edinburgh in 1850 and some hundred 'noblemen and gentlemen', including many distinguished foreign scientists, sat down to a 'sumptious dinner, combining the elegance of a great civic feast with the comfort of a private entertainment'. To accommodate the large party an elegant pavilion was erected in the garden 'the interior tastefully lined with pink and white cloth'. The decoration was provided by splendid exotics and the band of the 93rd Highlanders provided music. It was all a tremendous occasion and quite made the conference.

From the Minto House days Syme trained innumerable young men, many of whom were to make their mark in surgery or medicine. John Brown and Alexander Peddie, his two earliest assistants, were followed by those such as James Mackenzie, Thomas Annandale (1839–1908), John Chiene (1843–1923), Joseph Bell (1837–1911) and John Duncan (1839–1899) who all were notable surgeons in Edinburgh, by Edward Bickersteth (1828–1908) who became established in Liverpool, William Dobie (1828–1915) of Chester and a host of others. All remained loyal to their master and recognised the great privilege of having worked with him. Of his many assistants the one who stood head and shoulders above the others was Joseph Lister (1827–1912). It was Lister's happy and intimate association with Syme which led to the epoch-making career of the younger man with his contribution to surgical science, the greatest contribution of the century.

Joseph Lister had qualified from University College Hospital in 1852 and almost immediately had become a Fellow of the Royal College of Surgeons of England. It was at the suggestion of Syme's intimate friend Professor Sharpey that Lister came to Edinburgh in 1853 with the object of studying there for a month before undertaking a tour of the Continental schools. Syme was immediately attracted to the young London doctor and set him to work in his wards and to assist him in his private practice. Lister found in Syme's surgical practice much more interest and opportunity than he could hope for in London. Rather surprisingly he thought that Edinburgh, professionally, seemed a rather more peaceful place than London. He wrote to his father: [124]

> I shall not have, as in London to fight with jealous rivals, and contend or join ingloriously with quacks, but I shall be able, if all be well, to acquire a solid reputation in a legitimate manner, and then, if it seems desirable, move to London, and stand on my own ground there. I am by disposition very averse to quarrelling and contending with others. . . .

Lister soon learnt otherwise and his patience and tolerance were to be sorely tried in later years both in Edinburgh and London. But his path was made smooth in these early days and he quickly determined to extend his stay in Edinburgh over the winter to profit from Syme's teaching. He wrote enthusiastically: [125]

> Syme has his own views based on great experience with a sound judgement and a very original mind. . . . I am therefore quite satisfied that it will be well for me, if all go well, to spend the winter here even though my doing so should make my visit to the Continent exceedingly short.
> . . . I have nothing particular to say about myself, except that the stream of surgical instruction and of Syme's kindness continues to flow steadily and, if possible, increasingly. . . .

The projected month extended to eight years. Lister was soon appointed as a non-resident house surgeon to Syme and by the end of 1853 became a full house surgeon. The post was a junior one but Syme treated him as a favoured son and gave him special privileges and responsibilities. Soon Lister became an indispensable assistant and while working at his own experiments he began to edit many of Syme's lectures for publication in the *Lancet* and other journals. The death of Mackenzie late in 1854 determined his promotion to assistant surgeon in the Infirmary and settled that he should remain indefinitely in Edinburgh. Syme's friendship extended beyond professional matters and Lister, like other favoured assistants, became a constant visitor at Millbank. There he met Agnes, Syme's eldest daughter, and fell in love with her. They were married in the drawing-room at Millbank and part of the honeymoon was spent at Kinross with her uncle, David Syme, the Sheriff-Substitute of the county. In marrying one of another denomination Lister had to sacrifice his membership of the Quakers to which he was bound by a strong family tradition. He did this after much heart searching and later became an Episcopalian. It was an ideal marriage for Agnes proved a wonderful support in every way. The link with Syme was strengthened and the way was paved for Lister's appointment in 1860 as Professor of Surgery in Glasgow, where he evolved the antiseptic doctrine, and for his eventual return to Edinburgh to succeed his father-in-law in 1869.

Although Syme was so well known in Edinburgh as a surgeon he did not often participate publicly in affairs outside medicine. He took no active part in the general politics of the day although in medico-political matters he was often in touch with members of the Cabinet. Such interest as he had in politics was in support of the Liberal party. In the mid-century, Scotland was torn by sectarian strife and it has been noted how this had repercussions in University affairs. Syme made no public expression of his religious beliefs although his biographer Paterson describes his 'great veneration for religion' and considered that such feelings prompted his earnestness of character and a love for truth. The suggestion has been made that in his affiliation to the Church he showed the same tendencies as the Vicar of Bray but this perhaps should be discounted for it is known that for many years he was a regular and devout worshipper at St John's Episcopal church in Princes Street. His religious life was a private affair and he undoubtedly held deep and firm beliefs.

The picture is that of a man wedded to a professional life conducted in a prescribed routine. The daily task accomplished there was a retreat to the comfort and peace of his home and garden. The social circle was limited to long tried friends and those of his family. Pleasures were simple and confined to his garden and his long walks in the country. His practice was conducted in an orderly and punctual fashion and he was blessed with an exceptional memory which allowed him to fulfil his obligations without the promptings of a secretary. In his voluminous writings he had some assistance from Lister but most were achieved in his own hand. With his strong sense of duty, but perhaps with some degree of reluctance, he had often to break his formal routine and travel to London or elsewhere but his happiness lay in an ordered way of life in which his professional activities were clearly separated from his leisure hours. This existence was suited to his temperament and allowed him to achieve so much in his chosen profession throughout his whole life. There were no financial worries and the not inconsiderable fortune which he accumulated, as his will was to show, was invested securely.

Simpson led a very different life and pursued all sorts of general interests and enthusiasms. His domestic life was closely bound up with his professional activities for he conducted his practice from Queen Street.

The Simpsons had nine children who brought them great happiness but sorrows also. Margaret, born in 1840, died of diphtheria at the age of four. David, the eldest son, was born in 1842, qualified as a doctor and died in 1866. Walter, born in 1843, succeeded to the baronetcy. Mary died in infancy in 1847. Jessie, born in 1849, died shortly after David. James, born in 1846, was a chronic invalid all his life and died in 1862. William, born in 1850 and Alexander, born in 1852, survived into adult life. Eve, the youngest of the family, was born in 1854 and died in 1919.

Even in good social circumstances it was not uncommon in a large Victorian family for such a large proportion of the children to die young. The mortality rate in the Simpson family reflected the contemporary infantile and child mortality, particularly from infectious diseases. These tragedies were crushing blows to a man of Simpson's sensitive character and they induced periods of depression and an intense searching of the heart in matters of religious belief. Despite all this there was usually a background of great gaiety and happiness in the household. Somehow Simpson found time to play with his children, to read to them and to instruct them. Eve inscribes her biography to one who 'was not merely the best of fathers, but the best of men, and whose lessons of love will ever abide with me. . . .' His love for his own children was reflected in his intense compassion for other children who came to him as patients. When they grew up they never forgot his kindness and one recorded how Simpson was 'someone among the grown-ups we counted as one of us'. He had a remarkable facility for inventing exciting games and competitions and for interesting his own and other children in natural history or in antiquities. There was a round of parties at Queen Street, usually arranged on an impulse, in which adults and children joined. In particular there was a craze for acting and for 'tableaux vivantes'. On one occasion Simpson and a colleague brought down the house when they entered dressed as children and sucking oranges to enact the 'Babes in the Wood'.

The house was large but it had to accommodate not only the family and servants but also the practice. There were two consulting rooms and bedrooms were reserved for patients who came from afar and required observation or treatment. One or more assistants usually lived with the family and visitors were frequent. The establishment was really a mixture of a nursing home and an hotel.[126]

A constant stream of patients came to the house. The poor were seen on the ground floor by Simpson's assistants while private patients went up to a room on the first floor. At first there was no system and chaos reigned. Storer, a young American, recalled how he visited Simpson in 1853 to find 'the hall filled with women and many good ladies ascending the stairs'. No sooner had he arrived than Storer was asked to examine a lady from New York. Simpson in conducting his practice had no great respect for rank or position and if he had to descend to help his assistants the private patients remained kicking their heels upstairs. He ran his consultations like a clinic and as well as his assistants some students might be in attendance. Eventually some sort of order was achieved and the consulting hours were limited to the afternoon when patients, rich and poor alike, drew lots for priority and were marshalled in a dictatorial fashion by a succession of faithful manservants, of whom Jarvis was most successful in preventing Simpson from being imposed upon.[127]

Examinations were done rapidly, diagnoses established at once and treatment often instituted forthwith. The practice was not confined to obstetrics but patients came with all sorts of complaints. Simpson never regarded himself as a pure obstetrician but was prepared to cope with almost any medical or surgical problem. By 1850 he had such a reputation that he was swamped with patients who were confident in the belief that he and he alone could cure them. Some were referred from the Edinburgh practitioners but many came independently from all over the country or from abroad. These patients would take up residence in an Edinburgh hotel and some would cheerfully wait their turn for a consultation. Others were more peremptory and summoned the great man to them. Sometimes he went at once but the volume of his practice was such that there were many messages or letters complaining of his unpunctuality or his complete failure to visit. Some of Simpson's friends were so concerned about the reports of his carelessness in keeping appointments and in communicating with his colleagues that they wrote him long letters of warning and advice, in particular that he should keep an orderly appointment book! If he was careless in these matters at least it can be said that rich and poor suffered alike.[128]

There was a large proportion of the famous or the aristocratic for he was very much the fashionable doctor. He could gain the confidence of a duchess as easily as that of a Newhaven fish-wife. He was often called to the great houses of Scotland and England to assist at the birth of a child. He enjoyed such visits and never quite outgrew the pleasure which he, the 'poor baker's son', experienced from rubbing shoulders with the highest of the land. He returned to his family to regale them with the latest news of the fashions and customs of the aristocracy.

Simpson was so well known that Thackeray even brought him into a novel. His name appears frequently in memoirs and biographies of the period for if ladies of rank and education had not actually consulted Simpson they at least knew something of his methods. For example there was Effie, the young wife of John Ruskin, who was for long under his care. In her letters there is ample evidence of the trust she placed in Simpson. He understood her complaints, which may have been largely psychosomatic, and it is clear that she confided in him to a degree unusual at the time, (Simpson was often criticised for his frank methods of questioning his patients on matters which were thought almost too delicate for discussion). His advice that Effie should have a child, had this been possible to follow, might well have resulted in the salvage of the Ruskins' marriage. Effie wrote to a friend: [129]

> I quite think with you that if I had children my health might be quite restored. Simpson and several of the best medical men have said so to me. . . . I often think I would be a much happier, better, person if I was more like the rest of my sex in this respect.

To her mother she wrote in 1853: [130]

> I have been very fortunate about Simpson. . . . He came to me yesterday and again today. . . . He says that I am just in the same state as before but rather worse—the throat much swollen and the whole mucous membrane in a state of irritation. He says that I am to eat everything I like and to take some pills, to rub myself all over with olive oil at night which is to fatten me and when I am poorly to take Chloroform Pills instead of the liquid. . . . I never saw such a dear kind man as he is.

The suggestion that Mrs Ruskin should rub herself with olive oil draws attention to one of Simpson's favourite prescriptions. He wrote several papers on the subject of 'external oil-inunction'. This arose from a visit he paid to Galashiels where his friend Dr McDougall drew his attention to the healthy state of workers in the woollen factories as compared with other inhabitants of the town. It was the popular belief that the wool workers whose clothes became impregnated with oil were protected against lung and other diseases. It was customary even to put sickly children to work in the factories to improve their health. With his usual thoroughness Simpson made enquiries all over Scotland and confirmed that these beliefs were held in other wool manufacturing towns. From such observations he developed a régime of oil inunction and friction which he thought to be beneficial in a variety of conditions. His proof of the value of the treatment was not very convincing but it was a popular remedy and psychologically, at least, it must often have worked wonders.[131]

Most of Simpson's patients were women and there was, inevitably, a high proportion of the neurotic. He knew how to deal with them; he was not above employing his powers of hypnotism and many were dismissed with terse and simple advice. When neurosis was presented in the aristocracy this called for the utmost tact and diplomacy and a letter from his former assistant Priestley, working in London in 1867, shows us the kind of case that Simpson sometimes had to manage: [132]

> The Viscountess H——— . . . wants a child (£40,000 a year which goes if she has no child) . . . cannot be persuaded to give up her excessively gay life and give her body and mind some rest . . . during the London season she wears herself out . . . she actually shrivels up and the womb itself recurs to atrophy . . . she is not a safe patient to meddle with and difficult to manage when ill . . . a spoilt child in fact.

It was not just the crowd of eager patients which made Queen Street such a circus and the nearby cab rank the most profitable in Edinburgh! There was a continuous influx of other visitors; for Simpson's hospitality was proverbial. They came to breakfast, to lunch and, although he tried to keep the evening meal a family affair, they often stayed to dinner. Dr Pascale, of Italy, called one day and recorded: [133]

> The house of the celebrated doctor is, one may say, the temple of hospitality, and he does the honours with a touching solicitude, seconded by his excellent wife, whose engaging and agreeable manners call from all their guests respect and acknowledgement. It is not only on this occasion . . . that this temple is open to visitors, but every day of the year.

It is pleasant to find some mention of Mrs Simpson for she must have shown wonderful patience and skill in managing this erratic household. It seems unlikely that she ever had

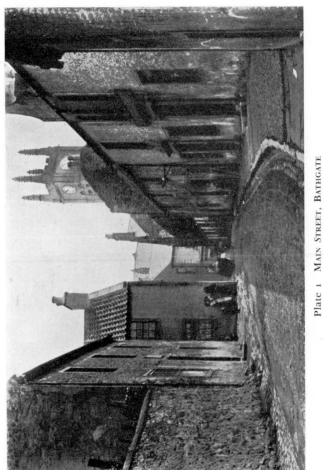

Plate 1 MAIN STREET, BATHGATE

Simpson was born in the house in the left foreground. This and the houses opposite have now been demolished (see reference 20, chapter 3).

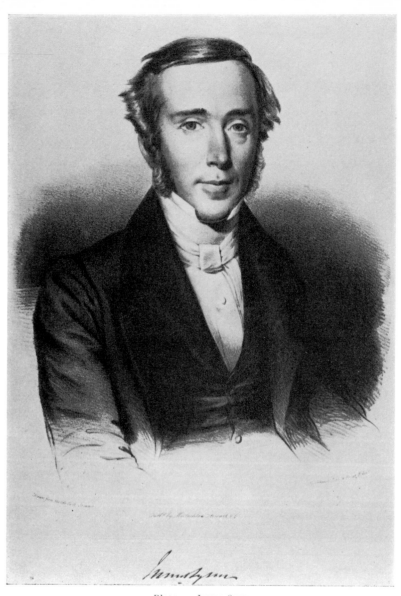

Plate 2   JAMES SYME
Aged about 45.

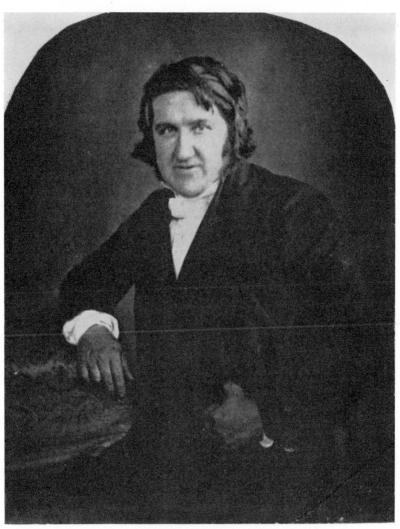

Plate 3   JAMES SIMPSON
Aged about 45.

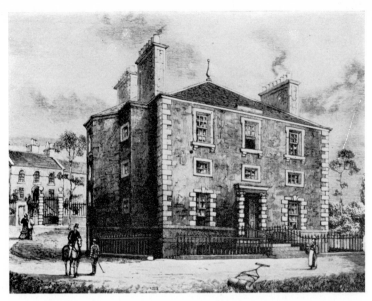

Plate 4 MINTO HOUSE
Syme's private hospital, sited on what is now Chambers Street and demolished about 1870.

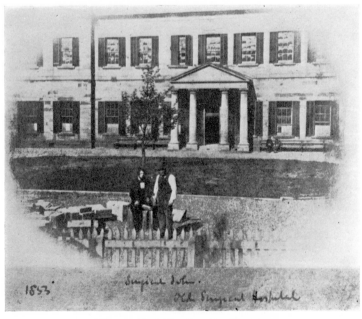

Plate 5 THE OLD SURGICAL HOSPITAL
The old High School was converted for use as a surgical unit of the Royal Infirmary in 1832. Syme did much of his work here and so also did Lister. The building survives as a University department unconnected with the medical school.

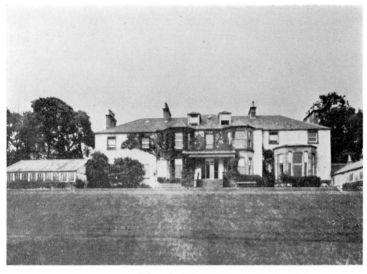

Plate 6   MILLBANK
Syme's country house at Corstorphine, then on the outskirts of Edinburgh.
The gardens survive but the house is replaced by a ward block of the Astley
Ainslie Hospital.

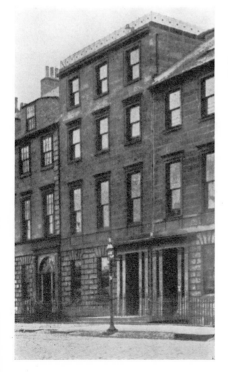

Plate 7   52 QUEEN STREET
Simpson's home from 1845 to
1870. The exterior stands unchanged today.

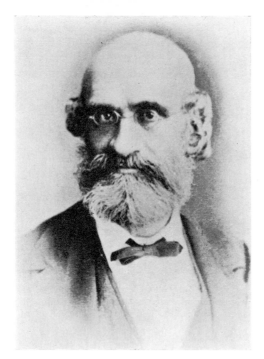

Plate 8   DR DAVID WAL.
Waldie suggested to Simp
the use of chloroform as
anaesthetic.

Plate 9
DR JAMES MATTHEWS DUNCAN
Duncan and George Keith
joined Simpson in the
historic trial of chloroform at
52 Queen Street on 4th
November 1847.

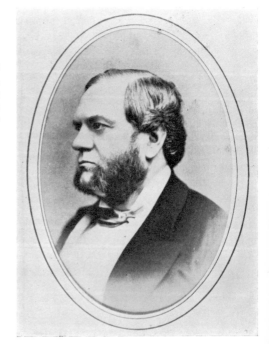

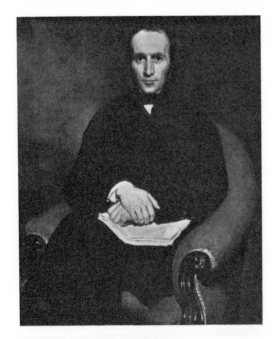

Plate 10   DR GEORGE KEITH
The third member of the chloroform party.

Plate 11
PROFESSOR JAMES MILLER
A close observer of Simp-
son's experiments and one
of the first to use ether in
Edinburgh.

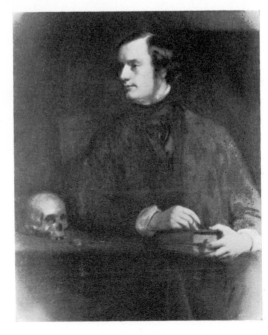

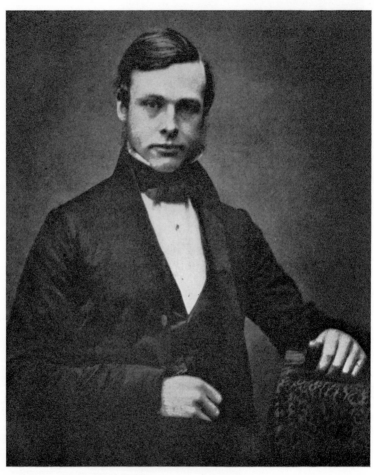

Plate 12 JOSEPH LISTER
Aged about 28. Syme's foremost pupil.

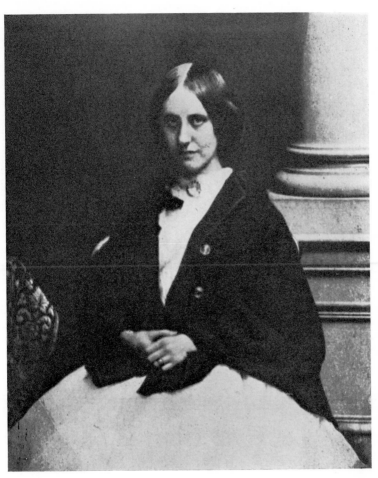

Plate 13   AGNES LISTER
Daughter of James Syme.

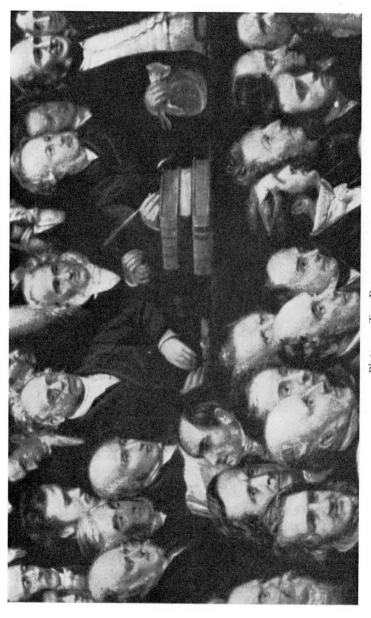

Plate 14   THE DISRUPTION

Part of the painting by Octavia Hill of the first Assembly of The Free Church in 1843. Simpson is in the left hand bottom corner. The artist made sketches at the event and com-

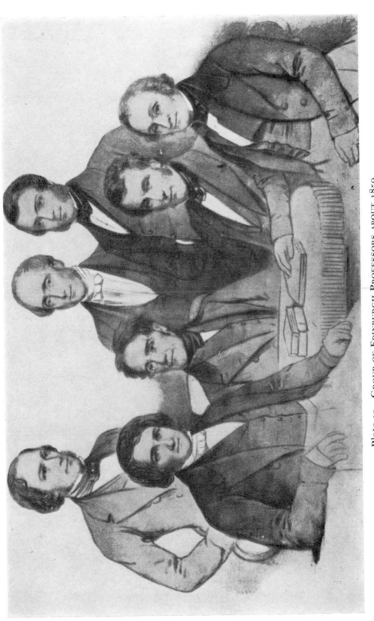

Plate 15   GROUP OF EDINBURGH PROFESSORS ABOUT 1850
Back row, left to right: Miller, Balfour and Bennet. Front row: Simpson, Jameson, Alison and Traill.

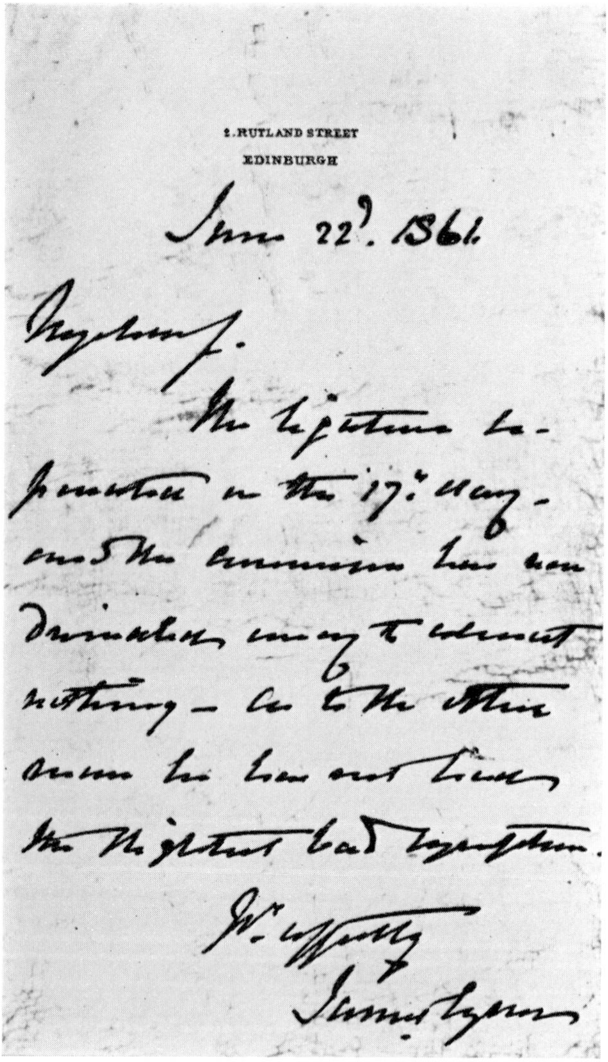

2. RUTLAND STREET
EDINBURGH

June 22d. 1861.

My dear Sir,

[illegible]

James Syme

Plate 16 Handwriting of Syme

Syme had two sizes of notepaper and usually filled one side of a sheet exactly in his orderly, succinct style.

My Dear Wells

  I hope you will kindly
excuse me ^writing^ & asking some
assistance from You, as
indeed I very much require
it. — You are almost a party
also in my present dusfer-
tunes, as it all d- seems,
originates in my publishing
the Clinical Lectures in

Simpson wrote his letters on notepaper of all kinds, in obvious haste, with
numerous corrections and frequent underlinings. No great skill is required
to contrast the characters of the two men from their calligraphy!

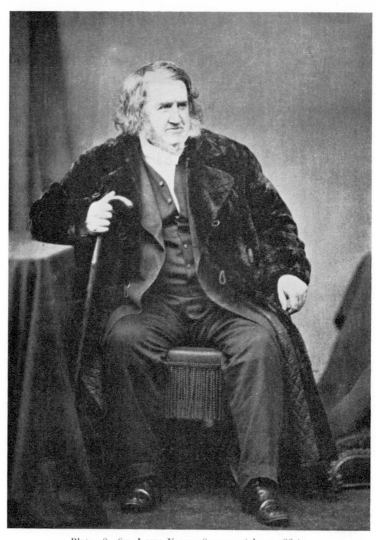

Plate 18 SIR JAMES YOUNG SIMPSON (about 1867).

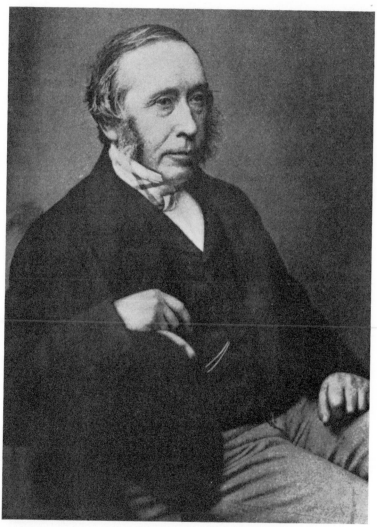

Plate 19 PROFESSOR JAMES SYME (about 1868).

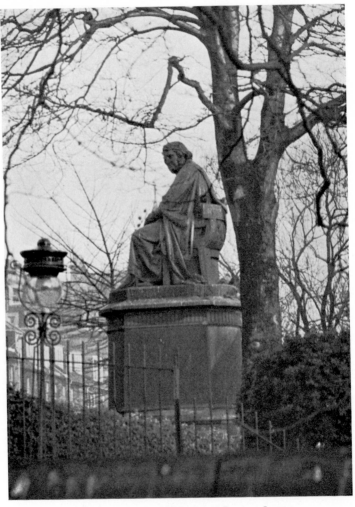

Plate 20   STATUE OF SIMPSON IN PRINCES STREET

There is some irony in that the photograph is taken looking up over
the wall of the small graveyard of St John's Church where Syme lies
buried!

the slightest idea how many people would sit down to breakfast or any other meal!

There were not only the doctors but there were antiquarians, writers, poets, artists and other celebrities. There were
not a few who came for their own ends, to seek patronage, to
try and interest Simpson in some wild-cat scheme or just to
borrow money. A description of a luncheon party in 1855
conveys some idea of life in Queen Street: [134]

> . . . with nothing in common save their wish to meet their
> host you find a company drawn together from every latitude
> and longitude, social and geographical . . . the grades and
> classes of eminence run through the whole gamut of social
> distinction, from duchesses, poets and earls, down to the
> author of the last successful book in cookery, the inventor
> of the oddest new patent, a Greek courtier, a Russian prince
> or a German count . . . Dr Simpson enters.
>
> With a few genial nods, shakes the hand to the nearest, he
> begins to despatch the coffee and roll put ready for him, while
> a brother professor at one ear propounds a question of Uni-
> versity discipline and a soldier just arrived from the seat of
> war is giving him, at the other, the anecdote with which before
> evening the doctor will, in abrupt episodes of consultation,
> have amused a hundred patients. In ten minutes the indefati-
> gable Professor is again professional . . . he disappears to the
> consulting rooms, or news comes by telegraph that some poor
> peasant's wife, in some far village, is in the dangerous stage of
> some medically interesting calamity. There are none-knows-
> how-many wealthy invalids waiting their turn but kindhearted-
> ness and the delights of a desperate case prevail, and the doctor
> is off across the Forth, and will not be back till midnight.

In fact there was a perpetual salon and no one of note who
came to Edinburgh could afford to miss seeing the Professor,
even although he might emerge with little more than a hand-
shake. Simpson loved meeting people and having quickly
discovered their interests extracted from them all the information he could to store in his massive brain for future
reference.

If a medical colleague arrived expecting a prolonged and
serious technical discussion he soon found his mistake. He
would at once be swept into whatever domestic or professional
activities were in train. Spencer Wells, then a young surgeon

on extended leave from the navy and eagerly seeking advancement as a consultant in civil life, gave an account of a hectic visit to Edinburgh at New Year in 1854: [135]

> The night was spent with Simpson, Priestley, and others, visiting the prison, whiskey shops and low haunts of that city! next day amongst Simpson's private and hospital work. At night Simpson entered into a learned discussion at the Royal Society on some of the Buddhist opinions and monuments of Asia compared with the symbols of the ancient sculptured 'standing stones' of Scotland. After the meeting Simpson drove him to a country house, the scene of the Ball in Waverley where patients were visited in the middle of the night: the house and grounds were seen by moonlight, and Edinburgh only reached early in the morning. That day Mr Wells did his operation in the Edinburgh Infirmary, and returned to London in the evening. Simpson having been in bed only two hours all this time—no uncommon example it was said of his marvellous activity and powers of work.

Simpson often took his guests round the sights of Edinburgh. His favourite conducted tour was to the old part of the city. He knew the dark and noisome closes of the High Street like the back of his hand, from the time he had been a dispensary assistant to Dr Gairdner. Even when he became the successful and fashionable consultant he often penetrated to the slums of the city to visit some poor woman with a complicated labour or serious disease. While he revelled in recounting the ancient history of Edinburgh to his visitors there was a philanthropic motive. He was greatly disturbed at the poverty and disease which was rife in the cities of Great Britain. Edinburgh was worse than most and Simpson did not hesitate to show the most sordid scenes as part of his campaign for reform. Dr Henry Lonsdale in his *Life of Robert Knox* gives a picture of the old town which he too knew well from dispensary practice: [136]

> The relapsing fever which prevailed as an epidemic in 1843 brought me in daily contact with the filthiest dens of the city and a population indescribably brutal and debased. Indeed in my walks through the worst parts of Paris, Rome, Naples, Stamboul and Jerusalem I do not remember seeing anything so shocking in the relations of humanity as was presented to me in the capital of Christian Scotland during the summer of 1843.

. . . Housed in the sunless and fetid alleys, or the worse tainted cul de sacs or 'closes', sheltering by dilapidated gables and sheds for cattle, or half smothered amid burrowed ruins and cellarage tenanted with rats and vermin, men, women and children huddled together in brutal fashion. . . . Human beings so lost to shame and natural feeling would have sold the corpse of their neighbours and as readily, that of their nearest relative, for a few bottles of whisky; nay their souls too, if anything like a profitable barter could have been done in that way.

Such conditions persisted for many years more and to Simpson were a matter of great concern, not only in their social implications but in so far as they determined the spread of so many diseases. There were enemies of Simpson who regarded his 'slumming' in the low wine shops and the brothels of the High Street as evidence of an immoral streak in his character. Similar aspersions were cast on William Gladstone when he, with completely philanthropic motives, consorted with the prostitutes of London!

There were frequent journeys for consultations far beyond Edinburgh. At first travel was entirely by coach or by private chaise. Although the coming of the railway simplified matters the carriages could scarcely be said to be comfortable. Simpson had his own inventions to ease his journeys. He devised a sort of deck chair which he placed between the hard seats of the carriage so that he could lie full length. He had a portable lamp to clip on to the carriage upholstery so that he could read or write at night. He became well known to the railway employees and if the waiting rooms were cold or closed he was always assured of a hot cup of tea with the station master or the guard. Details like these show his intense friendliness with his fellow men whatever their rank, a friendliness which was returned with the utmost affection.

If a journey was taken for professional purposes there was always time to fit in something extra: a friend to be visited, an antiquarian site investigated, some aspect of geology or of natural history to be studied. To the practitioner who called Simpson in consultation the visit was an event. The case seen and the treatment outlined, there was a meal and a long chat, often with reminiscences of student days. Dr Turner of Keith in Banffshire, remote and isolated from his colleagues, describes such a meeting. Simpson was in his district on a consultation and took great pains to contact Dr Turner: [137]

> I remember your face very well. We attended Knox together in 1831-32. . . . Our student days were, so to speak, lived over again: the College, The Infirmary and old Surgeon's Square supplying each its quota of pleasant memories. Isolated as I had in a great measure been, since beginning practice, from the men and things of the past, the after career of our Edinburgh coevals, teachers and taught, was little known to me: but Dr Simpson's information on this head, both for its content and its minuteness, was really amazing. . . .

More important Simpson had looked up Turner because he had read a recent paper of his on a subject of mutual interest. It was not just the friendliness of Simpson that counted but it was the encouragement he gave to this obscure country doctor.

Even the robust and energetic Simpson found the pace excessive at times. He had acquired a house, Viewbank, overlooking the sea at Granton and here he had some chance of a good night's rest away from the insistent demands of the night bell in Queen Street. The decision to move for a night or two to this retreat was taken at a moment's notice and on more than one occasion the long suffering butler was to be seen pursuing the family in a hired cab with the dinner which had already been prepared in the Queen Street kitchen. If Simpson did relax at Viewbank it was never for long and he always took with him a bag of books or the papers on which he was working. In the neighbouring village of Newhaven he took a great interest in the local community and had a high regard for this sturdy race of fishermen. Their wives came up to Edinburgh with their great creels of fish and their picturesque striped aprons and many were his friends and grateful patients.[138]

A wide circle of friends participated in the round of social activities in Queen Street. First of all there was a long succession of students and assistants, many of whom resided with the Simpsons for long periods and all of whom were welcome at meal times. A list of names would be lengthy, but mention may be made, in particular, of Robert Lawson Tait (1845-

1899) one of the many of Simpson's pupils who was to achieve greatness. Tait was born of very poor parents but with the help of scholarships at school and university soon attracted attention for his industry and ability. He became a protégé of Simpson and it seems certain that for a time he lodged with him at Queen Street. He remained one of Simpson's most staunch supporters and when he became a notable pioneer in abdominal surgery and was established as a gynaecologist in Birmingham, he never forgot the help and inspiration he had received from his chief. Tait had some resemblance to Simpson physically and in character he showed the same ruthless energy, combative spirit and originality. He too had a devotion to antiquarian studies. During Tait's lifetime and for long afterwards there were recurring suggestions that Tait was a natural son of Simpson. There is no real evidence for this although Tait himself, being of a mischievous nature, was not averse to fan the rumour by tousling his hair and mimicking the professor. When Tait died in 1899 his body was cremated in Liverpool but his ashes were laid in Warriston Cemetery close to the Simpson family grave.[139]

George Keith and Matthews Duncan, who collaborated in the discovery of the use of chloroform, remained for long as Simpson's private assistants. Both became estranged, Keith because of Simpson's quarrel with his brother Thomas and Duncan because he eventually became very much the rival of Simpson in obstetric work. Duncan was greatly disappointed when on Simpson's death he failed to obtain the Chair of Obstetrics and it went to Simpson's nephew. Thomas Keith was another assistant who became distinguished for his work on ovarian tumours and owed to Simpson all his early training. It was a great sorrow to Simpson that his friendship with the Keiths was broken because of a petty squabble over a matter of professional etiquette. Other assistants were Priestley, who later made his name in London, Watt Black, who edited Simpson's main writings on obstetrics, and the American, Horatio Storer, who on his return home incurred great enmity from his colleagues when he loyally championed the use of chloroform in obstetrical work.

Amongst the professors and teachers in the University, John

Reid, who when a student had taken the young Simpson under his wing, remained on terms of great intimacy. His story was a tragic one as after he was made Professor of Anatomy in the University of St Andrews he developed a malignant condition of the tongue. He died of this in 1846, after a distressing illness during which three ineffectual operations were attempted. For one of these he lodged with Simpson who cared for him devotedly. Simpson felt the death of Reid sorely and some there were who saw in this event a turning point in Simpson's religious life.[140]

Simpson had another intimate friend in Edward Forbes, a brilliant biologist, but he too died young, holding the Chair of Natural Science in Edinburgh for only a year. The rest of the professors were divided in their attitude to Simpson but he was on good terms with most of them apart from Syme and Alison. His friendship with Miller and Christison fluctuated according to events. Unfortunately there was always a nucleus of the professors only too willing to seize on any of Simpson's errors and to attack him openly or by more subtle means. His success in private practice undoubtedly antagonised many of his colleagues.

There were many friends in England as, for example, Thomas Spencer Wells. In 1850 Wells had, as already recorded, visited Simpson in Edinburgh and although an unknown young man was encouraged to demonstrate a new operation he had devised. Wells was one of many surgeons through whom Simpson kept in touch with London opinion. In July 1853 Wells, having just become editor of the *Medical Times*, wrote:[141]

> I hope our journal sometimes reaches as far North as Edinburgh. If so you will see that I have taken an early opportunity of advocating your claims upon the nation in connection with chloroform.
>
> I have not yet found a suitable house in town to commence practice in but I have a few patients to look after and trust you will not forget to send me some cases for plastic operations. . . . I don't want them to pay provided they don't put me to any expense.

Soon Spencer Wells became well known for his work on ovariotomy and was on equal terms with Simpson professionally. They remained close friends and it gave Wells great pleasure when Simpson received a baronetcy, for Wells had campaigned for many years for the readier recognition of doctors in the honours list.[142]

From his travels abroad and from his correspondence Simpson gained many foreign friends. Dumas, the distinguished French chemist, was in Edinburgh in 1847 and present at the first operations under chloroform. Retzius, the Swedish obstetrician, became a close friend and frequent visitor and was godfather to one of Simpson's children. Channing, of Boston, was one of many American admirers who took back to the New World news of Simpson's work. At times the drawing room was so crowded with foreign visitors that some likened it to the Tower of Babel!

Simpson, despite all his professional involvement and his university duties, found time for a multitude of interests outside medicine. From boyhood he showed an intense curiosity in every aspect of life. A scrap-book which he kept shows his extraordinary love of hoarding information. In this book are pasted poems, political cartoons, bizarre items of natural history such as the birth of a two-headed calf, medical news such as the account of spontaneous combustion in the corpse of a drunkard and even an article on the merits of ventilation of beaver hats! No little bit of information, printed or spoken, was despised and much was stored away in his capacious memory to be brought out in his sparkling conversation or applied in his scientific or other studies.[143]

There were some enthusiasms which did not last very long. In 1850 there was an exchange of letters with Keith Murray, the astronomer, from whom he sought advice on how to erect a powerful telescope with which to study the stars. There was a burst of activity during which the current textbooks on the subject were rapidly assimilated but quite suddenly the project was dropped![144]

A more detailed account must be given of Simpson's life-long interest, his antiquarian pursuits. It has been said that he took up this activity just after he became professor because many of his colleagues in the University despised him for his simple origin and for a lack of culture. In fact he was as well educated as most of his brother professors, although perhaps his knowledge of the classics was comparatively deficient. There is substantial evidence that although he was not unaware of the prestige associated with the production of original papers on subjects outside medicine and although he recognised the increased status acquired by membership of learned bodies, he took up archaeology and related subjects because he liked them. He found in such studies a relaxing hobby. He had shown from the start of his medical career an exceptional ability to seek out and marshal the history of his subject. He was well versed in early medical literature and his skill in this kind of historical research was readily applied elsewhere. He made his name in 1841 as a historian and antiquarian by the publication of an elaborate paper *On Leprosy and Leper Hospitals.* This was read to the medico-chirurgical society and when published as a pamphlet received great praise from all quarters. It is largely concerned with the incidence of leprosy in Scotland throughout the centuries. While the medical aspects are covered fully it is the intensive research from early parish records and from other medieval documents which impresses the reader. The work involved in the preparation of this paper must have been enormous. Considering that it was done in a relatively short time, while Simpson was so heavily involved establishing himself as a professor, it is almost impossible to imagine how he achieved it. The explanation lies partly in his facility in using the spare moments of life which most men waste, in his ability to seek out information not only in the libraries available to him but by contacting the right people and rapidly acquiring from them all the information possible. Much of his writing was done at night for his hours of sleep were short.

In 1872 John Stuart, secretary of the Society of Antiquarians of Scotland, collected and published all Simpson's archaeological essays. The list would have been impressive for a professional archaeologist. Some of the papers are brief but many are lengthy and learned reports. The topics range widely. He investigated stone-circles and other prehistoric remains such as the Cat-stane of Kirkliston, near Bathgate and the Calder stones, near Liverpool. There are ingenious pieces of detective work concerning medical practice in the

Roman armies of occupation in Britain. Early ecclesiastical ruins were of great interest to Simpson. Even the pyramids were studied in a paper entitled *Is the great pyramid of Gizeh a metrological monument?* Some people thought that Simpson was at times a bit dogmatic in his conclusions in all these matters and there was, for example, a heated argument over the latter paper, for in it he demolished the theories of Piazzi Smyth, the Professor of Practical Astronomy.[145]

In the preface to this collection Stuart describes it as being rather the 'exhaustive treatises of a leisurely student, than the occasional efforts of one overwhelmed with professional work'. Tribute is paid to the accuracy and sheer professionalism of Simpson's archaeological labours and how he stimulated interest in archaeology by his 'earnest truth-seeking spirit'.

All such work was a continuous source of pleasure to Simpson. If he travelled out of Edinburgh for any purpose he seldom missed the opportunity of visiting an important site, of calling on a local antiquarian or of appointing some agent to send him any curiosities from local excavations. Many other doctors combined their profession with that of archaeological research and letters flowed in to Simpson describing their discoveries or transmitting rare coins, fragments of pottery, seals or ancient documents.

In due course he was elected vice-president of the local society and in an address he gave very clear views of the purposes of archaeological study. He recalled the folk-lore transmitted to him in his youth by his parents and stressed how important it was that such information should be collected before it was completely forgotten.

Simpson's holidays were few and far between. After his operation in 1850 he took a prolonged trip to France, Germany, Holland and Belgium. Although he often set out with the intention of remaining incognito he could not resist visiting the hospitals and universities and it soon leaked out that the discoverer of chloroform had arrived. In Paris particularly he was greeted with great acclaim. There were several other continental visits, most of which were far from relaxing but involved rapid tours of hospitals and medical schools, intensive sight-seeing and meetings with fellow archaeologists. The last of these foreign visits was in 1868 when Simpson visited Rome and Florence. He was by then in poor health but determinedly viewed all the important antiquities and studied hospital organisations. He even found time to visit the grave of John Bell in the protestant cemetery and to arrange for its restoration. On all these visits he was besieged by patients and did many private consultations. Although he was invited to visit America by many of his friends there, he never undertook such a long trip. He was a poor sailor and disliked even the short sea trip to Ireland.

There were shorter breaks in the exhausting routine of Simpson's life when some distant consultation or medical conference was combined with a short holiday. Family holidays in the Isle of Man, often with the Liverpool Grindlays, were frequent but Simpson seldom joined his children for the whole of the period. On the impulse of the moment he sometimes rushed off for two or three days to the Lakes or to the Scottish Highlands. Usually there was a purpose such as an archaeological investigation following a report by a correspondent. It was typical that when in 1868 he went to Oxford to receive an honorary degree, ill although he was, he should tire himself out in coming home by Wiltshire so that he could rush around Avebury and Stonehenge, which he had long wished to view. He had a restless nature and once he had accomplished the object of his visit he was impelled to hurry back to his affairs in Edinburgh.

Simpson started his professional career heavily in debt. By about 1845 he was able to repay most of the various loans advanced to him. His private practice was soon such that there should have been no financial worries. Despite his early poverty he developed an extreme degree of carelessness with money. Fees were sought from his patients in an erratic fashion and there was no record of these transactions. It is said that his manservant had to go through his pockets at night to ensure that any money received was counted and deposited. At times he was extremely generous and either charged nothing or at a ridiculously low rate. A persistent financial instability was due very largely to two other things, his impulsive generosity and his gullibility over commercial adventures. Quite clearly it soon got around that he could

be touched for a loan by anyone with a story of misadventure
or hard luck. There are many pleading letters which suggest
that such debts were often unrepaid.

It was his commercial ventures which took him deeper into
the mire. It is not quite clear whether he sought to make a
fortune or that he merely loved the excitement of a gamble.
The latter explanation is perhaps correct for without his
commercial dealings he could have been assured of a steady
and lavish income. In his last years considerations for the
future of his family weighed heavily upon him. He wrote to
his son Walter in 1867: [146]

> I am in GREAT distress for —— and Co. hold that I am
> legally co-purchaser of the —— Works, though I repudiated
> the purchase weeks ago. They threaten, and will, I believe,
> take law steps in the matter. . . . You can easily imagine the pain
> I have felt for weeks past and this has aggravated it all, as the
> idea comes burning back on me by night and by day—that I
> have used you so ill, by squandering thus the money which I
> should have collected for you, as my heir. Often I wish I could
> unbaronet myself. But you must make your own fortune. I
> know you will forgive me, but I cannot easily forgive myself.

There are many such letters which show the tangle in which
Simpson found himself, the intense worry which he brought
on his head and the simple fact that he was no business man.

Through the Liverpool connection he developed interests
in mercantile ventures. He became the owner or part owner
of several ships and there was profit to be made either from
the merchandise carried or from the resale of the ships. One
at least, the *Araminta*, was lost but Simpson received £2,000
in insurance. All these negotiations involved very large sums
of money and it is uncertain whether or not Simpson eventually made a profit by them. At times the complicated business
between the Grindlays and the Simpsons led to family strife
and Mrs Simpson became at least temporarily estranged from
one of her brothers over a muddled transaction.

The most disastrous affair was Simpson's purchase of a share
of a sugar plantation in Tobago in 1859. Initially he invested
£5,000. A manager was appointed but he did not go near
the estate and left the supervision to an inefficient deputy.
In 1860 the sugar crop was a failure and there was a loss of

£3,400 of which Simpson had to pay half. It was not surprising that in 1867 Simpson revoked his interest and his losses, although they are not specified exactly, must have run into thousands of pounds.

The Tobago venture was by far the most costly to Simpson both in money and anxiety. But there were other investments which proved disastrous such as the Midcalder Mineral Oil Company in which Simpson in 1869 (perhaps in a desperate attempt to recoup his West Indian losses) invested £6,000.

Simpson's inventive faculty is revealed in his experimental work on industrial processes from which he hoped to acquire profitable patent rights. There was 'Simpson's Incomparable Anti-friction Lubricant'. By a few well devised experiments he proved that Rangoon petroleum was a far better lubricant for machinery than was sperm oil, commonly used at the time. He was very elated at this demonstration but when he tried to patent it he found that he had been forestalled. In 1867 he took out a patent for the manufacture of Trinidad pitch but there is no evidence that the process was successful or profitable. Perhaps most interesting of all is the 'provisional specification' in 1867 of an invention of a device to burn shale oil. Simpson suggested that if the oil was delivered in a fine spray mixed with air it could be ignited to produce light or heat. Nothing came of this projected patent and perhaps he could hardly have expected to lead in a field of engineering development in which there was great activity at the time. Simpson became, through family connections, heavily involved in the exploitation of the shale-oil and coal seams in the Bathgate district. While he may not have derived much financial benefit from these affairs, he must at least be credited with a remarkable knowledge of subjects quite outside his own sphere.

In all these erratic and expensive schemes Mrs Simpson was often involved, understandably in the family shipping business. It was perhaps tactful that it was in her name that certain transactions concerning chloroform took place. There had been a considerable outcry when the Americans tried to patent ether and if it had been known that Simpson was in any way connected with profit-making enterprises in the retail of chloroform there would have been trouble. Everyone

must have recognised, of course, that to Simpson the Edinburgh firm of Duncan and Flockhart owed their huge and
profitable turnover in the sales of chloroform which continued
for 50 years or more. Perhaps it was just as well that they did
not know that in 1848 Simpson arranged for a supply of
chloroform and of special bottles to be sent to Captain Neall
of the *Orpheus* in Leith Docks—for an outlay of £10 14s od.
The ship went to South America and Captain Neall sold
124 oz. of chloroform in Rio at a profit of £14! Mrs Simpson
and her Liverpool brothers were involved in this and the
venture seemed to interest them rather excessively. Perhaps
they hoped to open up a new and profitable export trade!
Robert Grindlay wrote to his sister Jessie in June 1848: [147]

> You seemed anxious to hear about your chloroform sent me
> by Mr ——. Neill says he sold it for about 4s. fl. oz. What did
> it cost and what was to be my share of the spec?—none of the
> money is yet remitted and I see the rate of exchange is falling
> daily so there will be a small loss there. . . .

It is all too clear that in his financial affairs Simpson became
heavily involved. All this must have been a great anxiety to
him and taken a toll insofar as his health and peace of mind
were concerned. His failures were the common knowledge of
his friends and when things went wrong there were many
letters of commiseration. To his enemies these activities were
examples of his unreliability and his profligacy. When, towards the end of his career, he was outvoted in the election
for the Principalship of Edinburgh University such matters
may well have been used against him.

There were literary interests of all kinds. Simpson knew
the novels of Sir Walter Scott well, discussed the latest of
Trollope's works with his patients, could quote the poet Burns
in the vernacular and correspond with Mrs Gaskell over the
true identity of George Eliot. Writers as far removed as John
Ruskin and Hans Andersen were entertained to dinner. To
this familiarity with the contemporary literary scene was
added a scholarly knowledge of ancient literature. Simpson
accumulated a large library and although medical works
predominated there were in addition many historical or antiquarian books of great value. He must have spent lavishly on
books. There is, for example, a bookseller's account of 1850

which shows his catholic tastes. £12 6s. 3d. was expended on the *Antiquities of Denmark*, the works of Thucydides and the novels of D'Israeli. Much of Simpson's valuable library was dispersed but a portion of it, bequeathed to the College of Physicians by Simpson's nephew, can still be seen.[148]

Like Syme it was inevitable that Simpson from his medico-political interests knew something of the general political scene. He had many personal contacts with the leaders of government over the Medical Reform Bill and during the Crimean War. He supported Gladstone in his candidature for the position of Chancellor of Edinburgh University. He was not the first (or the last) eminent doctor who thought he might enter the lists with the professional politicians. In 1867 he threw himself wholeheartedly into the campaign of his friend Pender who was seeking election for Linlithgow as a Liberal. Simpson's speeches were shouted down and harshly criticised in the press. Behind the scenes, however, he exerted great influence on all matters of medical and social reform.

We turn to the controversial subject of Simpson's religious activities and beliefs. These must be considered against the turmoil which overwhelmed the Scottish Church during Simpson's life-time. The two important developments in these sectarian dissensions were the Disruption from the National Church of Scotland in 1843 and the growth thereafter of the Evangelistic movement. When there was a separatist movement with the subsequent establishment of a Free Church, over matters of administration rather than faith, Simpson threw in his lot with the rebels. On the dramatic occasion when the majority of the ministers of the established church walked out of the Assembly Hall, thus sacrificing their manses and their stipends, Simpson, with many other lay members, is said to have joined the protest march. The complicated politics need not occupy us but there is some necessity to examine Simpson's private views and to try and assess the effect these had on his life and character.[149]

He was brought up strictly by his parents in the accepted and simple Scottish traditions and he entered manhood imbued with strong basic Christian beliefs. Duns devotes much space to the thesis that Simpson in his early adult life weakened in his religious beliefs and in later life was a con-

verted sinner who returned to the fold. The account is sentimental and there is the rather self-satisfied feeling conveyed
by Duns that he was largely responsible for leading Simpson
back to the straight and narrow path. Eve Simpson, who might
have been biased but was nevertheless very close to him, was
at pains in her biography to deny that Simpson underwent
a conversion from 'an unhappy, unthinking, godless man, careless of the Hereafter'.

An analysis of Simpson's spiritual struggle is not really very
difficult. He was typical of many overwhelmed by the scientific
discoveries of the age. The development of geological science
overthrew the simple chronology of the Old Testament. Darwin's theory of evolution was the greater blow to established
doctrine. Simpson with his analytical mind and his constant
endeavour to apply new ideas and discoveries, not only to
medicine but to the whole of life, must have gone through
a long phase of struggle and even torment. To him doubts
and criticisms of established religion must have had an impact
far greater than to others. Such doubts were inevitably increased when he found himself championing the cause of
anaesthesia against the fixed views of some of the clergy and
many influential lay people. This controversy alone forced
him to study the tenets of religion in great depth. Some of
his contemporaries with similar problems responded by becoming atheists and joined the very large group of Victorians
who discarded the beliefs of their fathers completely. Simpson chose otherwise and after much heart searching accepted
without question the basic teaching of the New Testament.
In time his beliefs were so strongly held that he felt it his
duty to do something to impress them on others. As a reaction
to all which tended to overthrow the teaching of the Church
an evangelistic or revival movement developed strongly from
about 1845 onwards. Edinburgh had its full share in this and
Simpson was caught up in it all. It was much to the advantage of the revival movement to have a national figure playing
a prominent part. He was pressed to speak from the pulpit
or at public meetings. Many of his addresses and his pamphlets survive. The titles and the subject matter may to some
degree repel us but these must be seen against the uneasy
background of the times. These public utterances created

an image of Simpson which was perhaps exaggerated but which survived long after his death. Not only did Duns over-stress this aspect of his character but there were other sancti-monious accounts. *Golden Vials Filled* by Barbour is one ex-ample and the Reverend Bullock published a similar eulogy in his *Leaves from Consecrated Lives.* While Simpson's in-volvement in this public witness of religion cannot be ignored, it need not be elaborated upon. It is simpler and probably correct to quote his own statement, 'I like the plain gospel truth and don't care to go into questions beyond that.' This was the way he was brought up and despite all the pressures exerted upon him he was able to make a compromise and it was in a simple faith that he died.

He felt greatly the loss of so many of his children in their early years. The final blow was when his son David died, just as he was entering a promising medical career and appeared to be the natural successor of his father in the Chair of Obstetrics. But as has already been suggested such losses were almost the expectation in a Victorian family. There are letters recording these family tragedies and their tone is exactly similar to those of so many other family letters in similar circumstances, deeply sorrowful but accepting the will of God unquestionably. It may well be that the loss of his friend John Reid had a great effect on Simpson. He saw Reid die at the height of his career and he knew of his heroic and resigned struggle against adversity. Reid also was fated to have a biog-rapher who went to great pains to show how the sinner had died repentant.

In his personal life it is clear that Simpson strove hard to follow the precepts which in his later years he proclaimed in public. He was a regular member of his church, at first the established body and after 1843 the Free Church. He became an elder of St Stephen's Church but he did not take up this office easily at the time because it demanded that he should subscribe to beliefs which he found difficult to accept. Increasingly over the years, in his addresses to his students, Simpson tried to impress on them the necessity for a Christian way of life. Perhaps in these later years some of his associates found his zeal oppressive, for there is ample evidence that he tried hard to influence those with whom he worked. With

some his purpose was achieved for on leaving him one of his
assistants wrote: [150]

> It is indeed with real sorrow that I think of going away from
> 52 Queen Street, and the kind things I have found there. To
> you I am and ever shall be profoundly grateful for all your
> exceeding kindness towards me. I thank you from my heart also
> for the matchless professional advantages I have enjoyed here
> during the last five years. Moreover, I came here dead in
> trespasses and sins, and God has been pleased in His mercy
> to meet and quicken me; and I bless you for having brought
> me to this my spiritual birthplace.

An account is now given of a curious sequence of events.
The story reveals some further details of the background of
Simpson's life and the undercurrent of slander and black-
mail which harassed so many an eminent Victorian! The
affair, as will be shown, may have had relevance to the intrigues which developed in 1868 during the election of the
Principal of Edinburgh University.

The volume of Simpson's writings was such that he was
very much in need of secretarial assistance. About July 1850
a Mrs Q. consulted Simpson professionally and she was under
his care for a prolonged period. Simpson soon discovered that
her husband was well educated and had, also, the then unusual
qualification of being skilled in shorthand. He seemed to be
just the man required and he was installed as a secretary. In
retrospect Mrs Q. claimed that the remuneration was meagre
and that her husband was grossly overworked. She wrote to
Simpson in 1854 concerning her husband's work: [151]

> After a month he wrote to you that he really deemed it deroga-
> tory to remain with you to be subject to the violence of your
> temper and the indignities offered. You apologised and advised
> him to study medicine as a means of increasing his value to
> you . . . the peculiar nature and mode of conducting your
> practice rendered it almost imperative to exercise your literary
> work in hours when the rest of the world were slumbering . . .
> not only have you had the six days but the seventh! I regret
> he should have aided you in breaking the Sabbath . . . he was
> under the delusion that in rendering you assistance he was
> indirectly benefiting mankind.

Quite clearly Mr Q. found that it was exhausting in the

extreme to work with Simpson and perhaps any secretary
would have found it so. Mr Q. continued, however, in his
somewhat nerve-wracking task until in 1853 a crisis occurred.
Mr and Mrs Q. were in financial difficulties and were heavily
in debt for some furniture they had purchased. Mr Q.
succumbed to the temptation of stealing (or perhaps only
borrowing) some money entrusted to him by his employer
for another purpose. Simultaneously his creditors had had a
summons issued. Simpson at once dismissed Mr Q. from his
service and advised him to flee from Edinburgh to evade
arrest. At first there were plaintive letters from Mrs Q.
admitting her husband's errors and even showing some gratitude to Simpson. Soon the tone of the letters changed and he
was accused of having acted uncharitably and of having defamed Mr Q.'s character. If this had been a simple matter of
dismissal of a servant for reasons thought by the one party
unfair, the whole business might have died a natural death.
There was, however, a further complication and although the
rejected Mr Q. disappears from the scene, Mrs Q. became
more and more of a trouble-maker.

As an obstetrician Simpson had his share of dealing with
the problem of the illegitimate or unwanted infant. In his
private practice, often amongst the aristocracy, there was occasionally an appeal to him to arrange for the disposal of a
child so that scandal would be avoided. There are several
records of such transactions showing that Simpson was well
accustomed to find foster parents and that he acted as the
intermediary who paid the expenses. In 1852 he persuaded
Mr and Mrs Q. (who were childless) to adopt a baby boy.
The mother of the child was unmarried and had consulted
Syme initially. Syme diagnosed a pregnancy and sent her to
Simpson. The identity of the mother is unknown but there is
at least a strong hint that she was well born. It is important to
note that Mrs Simpson knew all about the adoption. She
wrote to a friend in August 1852: [151]

> My account of a certain little boy will I think gratify you. Six
> weeks ago he was adopted—by a lady and gentleman without
> family. The only demand made by them was that the child
> should not be claimed after they made it their own . . . he
> has received the name of R.Q. and is a very fine looking child.
> They are not wealthy—Mr Q. is a man of University (I believe

Oxford) education—Mrs Q. has got an experienced nurse to
take care of him. . . .

At first the adoption went smoothly and both Simpson and
his wife took a great interest in the child's progress. When
Mr Q. was dismissed it was still necessary for payments to
be sent for the child's care. It is quite clear from subsequent
letters written by Mrs Q. that she, verging on paranoia and
religious mania, embarked on a process little short of black-
mail. The dismissal of her husband still rankled and over the
years she inundated Simpson with letters in which she demanded to know who was the mother of the child. She
assumed that he came of a good family and demanded that
the mother should take some responsibility for him by assist-
ing in his upbringing. To these requests Simpson remained
adamant. To an intermediary he wrote: [151]

> Sometime ago you wrote to me asking the name of the parents
> of the child whom Mrs Q. took home under the sole condition
> that he should not be taken back from her by his parents and
> that he should be entirely surrendered to her.
>
> It is unnecessary, I believe, to state to you that I would
> transgress the principles of professional honour most gravely
> if I complied with such a request. The secret could do no good
> to Mrs Q. or the child, as the mother is in poverty and the
> father (as she informs me) seems unable to aid the boy. Till
> the mother divulged it I believed the father was unaware that
> a child existed but the mother tells me she had an opportunity
> of telling him of it two or three years ago. Mrs Q. may find the
> parentage from other quarters—but she cannot hope possibly
> to extract it from me.
>
> But as you have written on the matter I venture to trouble
> you with it in totally another light.
>
> Mrs Q. has (the mother informs me) written Professor Syme
> on the matter. Mr Syme and I are not friends, not even on
> speaking terms, but he has (I learn) informed Mrs Q. that
> he called me to see the mother for the first time a few days
> only before the child was born—she (the mother) having come
> a long distance to be under Mr Syme's professional care for
> supposed dropsy. After the child was born I had to make all
> arrangements. . . .

Despite such replies Mrs Q.'s demands continued and there
were new accusations! She wrote to Simpson: [151]

Perchance had I wished to retaliate I might have whispered words into your ears respecting your domestic relations which would have brought the blush of shame quickly to your face by reminding you that the sparkling cup hath charms.

She elaborated on the suggestion that there had been riotous living in Queen Street. In fact there is good reason to believe that Simpson was the most temperate of men and it could be that Mrs Q. had heard reports of some of the anaesthetic investigations which had ended at times in uproarious scenes. There were implications too that Simpson by his actions was transgressing the Christian principles which he was publicly professing. But this was not all; for a new element entered into the correspondence. In 1866 she wrote as follows: [151]

Your words to me fourteen years ago 'Will you oblige me by taking a child of mine . . .' At first I thought you were joking still your voice and manner were unusually grave and on my looking up to you I shall never forget the deep crimson in your cheeks and in one second I felt we understood each other . . . my self possession left me for it is not a trifling incident in the life of any sensitive young woman to confront a really great man under circumstances so painfully humiliating: my first impulse was to assure you that the secret was in safe keeping, but a second look assured me that silence must be observed. . . . We stood spellbound neither uttering a word. . . . Why all this confusion if this child was nothing to you but simply the child of a stranger? . . . Again on my asking you something respecting the boy you stamped your foot, looked terribly angry at me and said 'I tell you I am not the father of the boy'.

To a man in Simpson's position the accusation that he was the father of an illegitimate child must have been alarming in the extreme. Professional etiquette demanded that he could not divulge the names of the true parents. Anyone who heard even a rumour of the affair might draw unfortunate conclusions from the fact that he had dismissed Mr Q. with some alacrity and encouraged him to leave Edinburgh. Simpson knew that already Mrs Q. had been in communication with Syme, with the Reverend Dr Guthrie and perhaps with others. He was all too aware of the readiness with which his enemies would seize on such scandal.

It must be apparent that Mrs Q. was unhinged in her mind. The circumstances under which the mother of the child came under Simpson's care are such that the accusation can be firmly dismissed. Further, as has been noted, Mrs Simpson was involved from the start in the arrangements for the adoption of the baby. There were many attacks on Simpson's morals before and after his death and this one was certainly malicious and quite unfounded.

Mrs Q. ended the letter quoted above with a final demand for information about the child's mother and with a postscript in capital letters 'IF I HEAR NOTHING—I SHALL BY TUESDAY SEEK INFORMATION THROUGH PROFESSOR SYME'. Whether she did or did not divulge her monstrous suspicions to Professor Syme or any other person is unknown. It can only be inferred that she may have done so and inflicted great damage on Simpson. There must remain the possibility that the rumours she initiated were used to his detriment in his candidature for the Principalship. In particular there is the rather sinister matter of a letter which Syme wrote when the election was in progress and to which reference will be made in a later chapter.

CHAPTER 9

Acupressure and Ovariotomy

I N the middle third of the nineteenth century in surgery,
in the words of Sir Frederic Treves, there was a 'change
from the mumbling obscurity of mediaeval dullness into
the clear light of a precise science'. While the development
of general anaesthesia, in which Simpson played such a great
part, was of great significance, it was Lister's introduction of
the antiseptic method which finally opened the way to the
whole range of modern surgery. Other important new ideas
were, however, exploited about this time and some were
carried to near perfection.

It has been shown that to Syme new ideas were often suspect. A review of one of his books in 1862 is probably just in
its appreciation of this point: [152]

> Not seeking to establish grand theoretical ideas or ascend to
> those lofty heights of generalisations where feebler brains have
> not infrequently become giddy and resolutely turning away
> from those hardy speculations which are apt to seduce even
> men of superior vigour, Mr Syme's claims to our respect
> depend on the application to practical purposes of old fashioned
> but thoroughly established principles.

He certainly made for himself a reputation of extreme conservatism in surgical practice. In 1862, when he was made
chairman of a national committee to adjudicate on surgical
instruments, a contemporary observed: [153]

> he would well condemn everything . . . he who boasts that a
> knife, an artery forceps, a saw, a bone snipper and a catheter
> are all the machinery of scientific surgery.

Such simplicity had its roots in Syme's early training in a
school which emphasised the importance of sound anatomical

knowledge, the necessity of speed and the acceptance of set rules and techniques of operating and after care. The surgery of the pre-anaesthetic period, although it might appear brutal at times, could be and was, in the hands of an expert like Syme, carefully planned and admirably executed. It says much for Syme that he adapted himself remarkably well to many of the changes and challenges in his life-time. He accepted, after cautious trial, the benefits of general anaesthesia. He appreciated in his last years that Lister's work heralded a new era in surgery and this was when many of his colleagues, including the younger men, opposed Lister. That Syme supported two such important advances in surgery balances to some extent his rather conservative attitude towards other innovations.

Simpson in contrast showed a far greater readiness to explore new ideas and to discard the old. When Syme talked of those who became giddy with new speculations he was, of course, attacking Simpson more than any other. If prejudice or dogma was attacked by Simpson he was frequently accused of rushing to conclusions or of applying theory to practice prematurely. However, in comparison with most of his contemporaries, he almost invariably presented a well supported case for any change.

Syme, the 'pure' surgeon, was thus extremely wary of entering any new field. Simpson, maintaining throughout all his life an interest in the whole of medicine, produced more original ideas in surgery than did Syme, the specialist. Simpson's extraordinary capacity for hard work, his genius for invention and his intense curiosity are readily admitted but he was prepared to exploit new weapons such as microscopy and animal experiment while Syme scorned such things. The contrast between the two men is brought out by tracing their interventions in two great surgical controversies of the time. In both of these is reflected the history of the rapid expansion of surgery in the nineteenth century. The first argument involved Simpson's presentation of a new way of controlling bleeding vessels during operations, namely acupressure. The second concerned the propriety of the operation of ovariotomy.

As a technique acupressure was a failure and is now largely

forgotten. What should not be forgotten is that in his work Simpson is revealed at his best as a thinker and an experimentalist. The subject was tied up with all the wider problems of wound healing and wound infection and involved the basic principles of operating technique. It is almost ironical that Simpson the obstetrician and physician saw such problems so much more clearly than Syme the surgeon. It is not surprising that by daring to challenge the established ideas on surgical technique, Simpson incurred the enmity of Syme to a degree unparalleled in their earlier feuds.

In surgery the effective management of bleeding vessels has always been of great importance. When major surgery was limited largely to the amputation of limbs, and when these operations had to be done with great speed, the surgeon acquired exceptional dexterity in the control of the severed ends of large arteries and veins. Originally there was a crude technique of cauterising bleeding vessels with a red hot iron, a practice which was not only inefficient but which must have struck terror into the heart of the patient. John Bell wrote of this barbarous custom in his *Principles of Surgery*: [154]

> The horrors of the patient and his ungovernable cries, the hurry of the operator and assistants, the sparking of the irons and the hissing of the blood against them, must have made terrible scenes: and surgery must, in those days, have been a horrid trade.

Ambroise Paré in the sixteenth century introduced a more humane technique which transformed surgery. He showed an unusual defiance of mediaeval dogma. His own words, words which must have appealed greatly to Simpson, may be quoted: [155]

> For antiquity and custome in such things as are performed by art, ought not to have any sway, authority or place, contrary to reason, as they oft times have in civill affairs: wherefore let no man say unto us that *the ancients have always done this*.

Paré was a military surgeon and at the siege of Danvilliers in 1552, he defied surgical convention and discarded the cautery. The first use of his new method of dealing with the bleeding points in amputation is described as follows: [156]

There was a culverin shot pass'd atraverse the tent of M. de

Rohan which hit a gentleman's leg, which was of his trane: which I was fain to finish the cutting off, *the which was done without applying hot irons*. . . . The campe being broken up I returned to Paris with my gentleman whose leg I had cut off. I drest him and God cured him. I sent him to his home merry with a woodden leg and was content, saying that he escaped good cheape, not to have beene so miserably burnt.

Paré introduced the simple expedient of ligating vessels with thread. He passed a ligature by an instrument called the 'Crowe's beak' and strangled the vessel directly by the knot. Alternatively he used a needle and brought the ligature out through the skin to be tied on the surface over a 'bolster'. It was more than 100 years before this simple expedient was generally accepted by surgeons for there was a bitter rearguard action in support of the old methods.

Up to 1850 a wide variety of materials and instruments were devised to perfect the art of ligation. It was customary that on amputating a limb the surgeon would have his assistant control the bleeding point with his fingers or with a simple instrument known as a tenaculum and, later, the catch forceps invented by Liston. The assistant's skill was measured by his speed in seizing the spouting end of the vessel so that the surgeon could readily pass a ligature to obliterate it completely. Most surgeons favoured silk or pack-thread but a few used more unusual materials such as crude catgut (which was first suggested by Physick in America in 1822) or strips of chamois leather. If a large vessel was tied it was usual to leave the ends of the ligature long and to bring them out through the wound. In favourable circumstances the long ligature detached itself weeks after the operation without incident, but more often the long strands of what was inevitably an infected material caused a discharge of pus and considerable discomfort to the patient. At the worst, and not infrequently, infection in the vicinity of the ligature involved the vessel, the knot disintegrated and haemorrhage ensued which might be fatal. Smaller vessels were sealed by crushing with a crude form of artery forceps or by 'torsion', whereby the vessel was seized by forceps and simultaneously twisted and crushed. The methods were by no means reliable but most surgeons thought them the best available and accepted the hazards.

The use of the long ligature was so firmly established that many surgeons had come to regard it as beneficial. They did not expect wounds to heal without inflammation and the long ligature was thought to provide an effective drainage track for the foul discharge which so often collected in the wound. Most surgeons trained before 1850 were very reluctant to abandon this well tried technique.

Although before 1850 there were many sporadic attempts to achieve primary wound healing or healing by 'first intention', it was generally taught that this ideal was impossible. Most innovations involved new rituals of wound dressing but a few surgeons appreciated that simple cleanliness of their instruments and hands did something towards improving their results. Some tried to solve the problem by leaving wounds open; washed them out with water and closed them a few hours later. Others made no attempt to close their wounds but packed them with materials such as 'charpie', which was a particularly septic plug made of scraps of old linen. Sepsis did not perturb surgeons unduly since they recognised that if a lot of pus was localised in a wound and if this eventually discharged there would be, in many cases, complete if slow healing. For the patient the healing process was a weary business with the frequent painful removal of adherent dressings, a foul and persistent discharge and, not infrequently, a slow decline from toxaemia and loss of blood. In many cases, particularly in conditions of excessive crowding in filthy wards, a wound infection did not remain localised but caused death by a rapid spread of the process. The major scourges were listed as erysipelas, septicaemia, pyaemia and hospital gangrene. The pathology of such processes is now easily understood in terms of bacterial infection but before Lister's time was inexplicable.

Syme was all too aware of these terrible complications of infection. Like any other surgeon he did many an operation which at first promised well and then ended in disaster. He had, until late in his active career, the same confused ideas about inflammation as most of his contemporaries, attributing wound sepsis and its complications to hypothetical mechanisms such as 'constitutional irritability', 'local excitement of the part' or 'sympathy'. His attention was directed almost entirely to principles which would aid 'resolution'. Despite his early rejection of the excessive use of venesection, he continued to advocate a limited use of this long accepted therapy believing that in inflammation engorgement of the tissues with blood was deleterious. He was a strong advocate of local bleeding by leeches, scarification of the skin and cupping. He relied greatly on traditional methods of influencing the general functions by lavish use of purgatives or of drugs which made the patient sweat profusely. He applied counter-irritants with enthusiasm. He thought there was merit in the ancient Chinese method of acupuncture in which inflammatory reactions were treated by the insertion of long needles. Although there is little in his earlier writings to suggest that he had firm ideas as to how the septic complications of wounds could be prevented, he has been credited with having gone further towards an insistence on general cleanliness than did most of his contemporaries. Some have considered that in his techniques he laid the foundations of aseptic surgery but there are no real grounds for such a sweeping assertation. He rebelled against the over tight suturing of wounds and their tight compression under layer after layer of dressings. In amputations he followed the practice of Alanson, suturing the skin flaps lightly and applying the simplest of dressings. For a while he was enthusiastic about the repeated application of cold water dressings, which must at least have been comforting to the patient. It was to be many years before he even considered discarding the long ligature, but he may have diminished some of the complications associated directly with septic ligatures by using a fine waxed silk which was probably less irritant and less infected than the coarser and dirtier materials employed by others. In his last years it was the close contact with Lister which stimulated the older surgeon to look afresh at the problems of wound healing. Syme's influence, however, in this important field was largely indirect and it was Simpson who made a positive attack on the problem.

Simpson did only a limited amount of surgery compared with Syme. In his early years he had some experience of operations such as amputations. This and his intensive research into the mortality rate of amputations after the introduction of ether must have impressed on him the terrible mortality and morbidity of surgical operations. He saw the problem from a very broad angle and the extremes of his interests are shown in his research on acupressure and in his later work on the broader subject of 'hospitalism'. As an obstetrician and gynaecologist his operating was usually restricted to minor and local procedures in the accepted province of the specialty. He was not averse, however, to occasional excursions into other fields to remove external tumours or to operate for breast conditions. He did a few abdominal operations such as ovariotomy, as will be recorded.

There is no positive information about Simpson's technical skill as a general surgeon. If the harsh criticisms of some of his colleagues, Syme in particular, are accepted then there is at least a hint that when he went outside his specialty he was deficient. Such a suggestion must be looked at guardedly for it may well have arisen largely from the feeling that Simpson dabbled in surgery and that he should have confined himself entirely to obstetrics. Such criticisms were not unusual and for many years arguments raged in London and elsewhere as to the right of the obstetrician to perform major surgery, particularly in the abdomen. It is interesting to note that most foreign commentators regarded Simpson primarily as a surgeon. Perhaps it may be hazarded that temperamentally he was not well fitted to be a surgeon, that he might have been lacking in patience and in too much of a hurry to operate. It is recorded, however, that he had the most sensitive hands and that he was unsurpassed at some of the more delicate manipulations of obstetric work. Whatever Simpson's merits as an operating surgeon his work on acupressure shows him as a surgical thinker far superior to most of his contemporaries.

With his early study of pathology, his intense powers of observation and his remarkable flair for sifting the work of others Simpson had the great essential of the scientific worker, a prepared mind. It was a very simple observation which initiated his interest in wound healing. In his own field one of the biggest technical problems was the management of the condition of vesico-vaginal fistula. This was common after complicated childbirth and to relieve a patient of the consequent distressing effects of leakage from the bladder was the ambition of every surgeon. Such operations were usually attended by failure until in 1852 the American, Marion Sims, achieved some success by a method of closure of the hole in the bladder by metallic sutures. Simpson at once appreciated that here was the unusual circumstance of primary healing achieved in conditions which seemed completely inimical to success. He deduced that if an operative wound, often closed in conditions of established sepsis, would heal while subjected to the irritation of urine, there was surely special merit in metallic sutures.

It was not until 1864 that he embodied all his thoughts and experience in a large volume *Acupressure: A new method of arresting surgical haemorrhage and of accelerating the healing of wounds*. It is important to record the second part of the title for the work has been too often discussed as an exposition of a somewhat cranky means of controlling bleeding. It is, in fact, one of the most intelligent studies of the problems of wound healing to be published before 1867, when Lister announced his discoveries.

In his presidential address to the Medico-Chirurgical Society in 1853 Simpson gave an early indication of the work in which he was engaged. The paper was *On the modern advancement of Physic* and in it he reviewed recent developments in both medicine and surgery in a masterly fashion. In referring to the use of ligatures in the control of bleeding he accepted that Paré's discovery was of great significance but he added: [157]

is it not possible that surgery . . . finding some more advanced means to do without the irritation of a permanent ligature— may yet save the sides of the wound from the presence of any foreign body whatever within it . . . and thus add greatly to the chances of its speedy union by adhesive instead of suppurative inflammation?

He had already embarked on an elaborate series of experiments and observations. As always he sifted all the available writings on wound suture and wound healing, with particular reference to the use of metallic sutures. He corresponded with chemists and metallurgists concerning the properties of different metals. A mass of information was collected and published in a long series of papers until he finally collected the whole substance in his book in 1864. The first important article was in the *Medical Times and Gazette* of 1858 *On the use of metallic sutures and metallic ligatures in surgical wounds and operations.* He listed the wide variety of materials which had already been tried, such as silk, flax, pack-thread, catgut, leather and tendon material. He gave a long historical review of the use of metallic sutures, recording that Hippocrates had recommended golden thread and that in the earliest times silver wire had been used in hernia operations. Between 1830 and 1850 there had been a wave of enthusiasm for the use of metallic sutures in all kinds of operations. Morgan and Bransby Cooper in London had used platinum wire for skin wounds; in Paris Dieffenbach, the pioneer of plastic surgery, had used leaden threads for cleft palate operations. To Simpson the most significant advance was Marion Sims' use of silver wire for vesico-vaginal fistula, a technique taken up with success by Spencer Wells in London and by Simpson himself in Edinburgh (although he preferred iron wire).

It remained to prove that metallic sutures were associated with better healing than occurred with silk and other commonly used materials. In the second part of his paper Simpson propounded his 'Law of tolerance for living tissues for the presence of metallic foreign bodies'. There was a mass of experimental work and he chose the pig as the most suitable animal. With the help of two assistants, Edwards and Murray, he implanted various metallic sutures and proved that silver and iron gave the least reaction. He did a more important experiment, the full significance of which he could not grasp because he was unaware of the rôle of bacteria in infection. He implanted in one side of a pig the thread sutures from an infected wound and on the other side he implanted new silk thread. The dirty material soon produced a gross carbuncle and the control of clean thread produced only minor and delayed infection. His experimental observations were applied in humans and soon he reported, for example, the primary healing after a breast operation where platinum wire was used to close the wound.[158]

His arguments were reinforced by citing the well recognised tolerance of the tissues for bullets or other metallic missiles. He observed also how when the women of certain primitive tribes beautified themselves by inserting metal ornaments under the skin these foreign materials were not expelled. He quoted numerous observations by others, including Syme who in his earlier years had performed an important series of experiments on animals in an attempt to elucidate the problems of bone growth. Syme had inserted metallic plates in the tissues and had found that these were well tolerated.

Simpson carried his ideas about metallic sutures very much further than just to advocate their use for skin closures, which after all had already received some general acceptance. Quite simply he attributed most of the complications of wound healing to the use of silk and similar materials. He believed that he could apply the lessons learnt in his experimental work so that the surgeon could at last hope for primary healing with some consistency. He maintained that silk: [159]

imbibes animal fluids into its substance: and these dead fluids speedily decompose and render the threads morbidly poisonous and irritant agents to the contiguous living tissues . . .

. . . ligature threads become in a few days so loaded with irritant matter that when taken out and buried at that time in the depths of recent wounds in other animals they, as a usual effect, quickly incite in the tissues around them suppurative and sometimes furunculoid inflammation.

From such premises it was readily argued that any silk ligature inserted in a wound was a source of suppuration with all its potential risks. If, as in fact was usual, such deep ligatures crushed the cut ends of blood vessels then there was the additional hazard of implanting in the wound small fragments of dead tissue (the stumps of the blood vessels). There were plenty of authorities to quote concerning this point. Spencer Wells, for example, had written, 'Every surgeon knew that the part of the artery beyond the ligature must be killed by it and a piece of sloughy tissue cannot do any good when confined amid the living tissues of the body.' In more picturesque language Simpson affirmed that surgeons in ligating vessels with silk or other such materials 'were placing some minute morsels of dead flesh into the raw cavities or upon the raw sides of all their large wounds'. Further if the ligatures were left long the surgeon was in fact employing a 'seton', a device which was intended to produce suppuration and to delay healing.

His solution was to discard the use of buried ligatures of irritant materials like silk and to devise a method of control of bleeding vessels which eliminated, or at least diminished, damage to the vessels. This was the basis of the new technique to which he gave the name acupressure.

He announced his discovery to the Medico-Chirurgical Society in October 1858. He demonstrated how he had obliterated the carotid artery of a horse by the use of iron pins instead of ligatures. (Unfortunately we have no details of how he succeeded in conducting such a hazardous operation on a horse, but almost certainly chloroform was given.) A year later he made a much fuller communication to the Royal Society of Edinburgh and described the application of the technique to humans.

The principle was very simple. A long steel pin was passed through the tissues close to the artery or vein in such a way that it compressed the vessel; in Simpson's words just as 'we fasten the stalk of a flower in the lapelle of our coat by a pin'. A variety of devices were developed to keep the pin in position. It was retained just long enough for the vessel to become obliterated by adhesion and clotting. The pin was of iron or steel. It was reasonably clean if not completely sterilised and it was relatively non-irritant to the tissues. The extremity of the vessel beyond the site of obliteration did not slough as would happen with a septic thread ligature which crushed the stump. The pin was removed in 24 to 48 hours and so no foreign material was left in the depths of the wound. The chances of healing without suppuration was therefore much improved.

The placing of these needles was admittedly tricky but Simpson soon collected evidence that even the large arteries of the limbs could be controlled in this way. He was at a disadvantage for he was restricted to some extent in his own practice of operative surgery. He had to persuade his colleagues to use the method for amputations and other major procedures which offered a real test. In Edinburgh he gained a few supporters such as Handyside but in general the surgeons there were against him. Elsewhere in Scotland, Pirrie of Aberdeen and Greig of Dundee took up acupressure with enthusiasm. In England there was at first support from Spencer Wells in London and from his former assistant Lawson Tait, now a young and progressive surgeon in Wakefield. Lawson Tait had as a student worked under Simpson and done animal experiments at his direction. He published an article, while he was still a student, in which he courageously refuted the theories on arterial pathology held by an eminent foreign professor.[160]

Simpson conducted a prolonged and detailed correspondence with his friends and from them he collected an appreciable amount of evidence that acupressure was feasible, reasonably safe and it favoured rapid wound healing. Typical is a letter to Greig in January 1860:[161]

I am delighted to hear that you are getting on so excellently with acupressure. . . . What a curious generation of men surgeons in general are! If they were told for the first time that some barbarous races . . . after amputating legs or arms, placed a series of small dirty setons between the sides of their wounds and anchored these setons in the very depths of these wounds to bits of dead flesh, they would deem the practice most strange and savage. Yet the ligatures are after all, truly small decomposing setons, fixed to dead bits of arteries. Some, however, of my surgical friends here stoutly maintain that these setons and sloughs are very sanitary adjustments in wounds. . . .

In London the technique did not really catch on although Spencer Wells, now a surgeon of rising reputation and influence, was at first enthusiastic. He not only employed it but as editor gave Simpson considerable space in the *Medical Times and Gazette* to publicise the new discovery. Simpson wrote to Spencer Wells in 1860:[162]

. . . Please keep a page alive in this next No., and I will send you a paper—not a lecture on 'Acupressure in Amputations' with details of four cases of it on the leg, arm and foot. I have not got a word written; but will strive to do so tomorrow or Friday.

. . . Acupressure goes ahead. Dr Greig of Dundee has used it. . . . He doubted entirely about the 'thing' (as he termed it). His first trial of it upon the living subject amazed and converted him. Now he prophesies it must come into general adoption.

Simpson had no illusions about the opposition he would encounter. He knew from his experience with chloroform that a new idea in surgery or medicine would inevitably be opposed with vigour and vehemence. He knew that it was many years before Paré's advocacy of the ligature was accepted. He was cautious in his forecasts for he wrote: [163]

> I venture upon a prediction that within the next two or three generations—operators will have ceased to implant systematically, with arterial ligatures, small dead sloughs and irritating setons . . . and will arrest their haemorrhages by acupressure in some of its discovered or discoverable modification—or it may be by some other haemostatic means even still more safe and simple.

To Simpson acupressure was perhaps more important even than his discovery of the use of chloroform. He firmly believed that if acupressure was accepted surgery would be revolutionised and that his name would be remembered for this more than anything else. He devoted many years towards its perfection and its defence against all critics. It was perhaps the biggest disappointment of his life that he must have realised just before he died that acupressure was seen as but a transient novelty and that it would have no real place in surgical history.

Despite all his efforts acupressure never really became popular. Although Pirrie of Aberdeen continued to advocate it for many years most other surgeons discarded it after a few attempts. It took Simpson a long time to collect a respectable total of major amputations done by his supporters. He at least was well satisfied that primary healing was the rule and that complications were few. The medical press, at first tolerant and even optimistic about the success of acupressure, soon dismissed it as a nine days' wonder. In 1864 one reviewer wrote 'we must make allowances for the parental affection which Dr Simpson must naturally be expected to feel towards his own offspring'.

From other quarters there were more bitter criticisms and

in Edinburgh it was Syme who led the attacks. He considered
that Simpson was once again interfering in a field which
was not his own. Why should a mere obstetrician dare to
instruct surgeons in the basic techniques of their art? In
February 1860 Simpson wrote to Spencer Wells: [164]

> In our Infirmary here Mr Spence amputated twice yesterday
> —but of course he would not use acupressure 'a suggestion
> of a physician—Bah!' Nay Mr Syme, Mr Spence and Mr
> Gillespie have actually given in an application to the Managers
> of the hospital to prevent me operating on vesico-vaginal
> fistulae and in other cases of obstetric surgery. This is their
> answer to the proposition to use acupressure instead of liga-
> tures! But it is too late to stop acupressure now. . . . The
> Managers have summoned the surgeons to come before them
> tomorrow and state their case. I have two cases of vesico-vaginal
> fistulae going out this week cured at the first trial. One of
> these patients was in the surgical wards eight years ago and
> operated without success by Mr Syme. She has it appears been
> cured at an inopportune time, as her cure will be one of the
> grounds of complaint.

The battle was joined in no uncertain way and this
attempt by the surgeons to restrict the surgical activities of
the obstetricians worried Simpson greatly. Two days later he
wrote to Spencer Wells in some desperation: [165]

> I hope you will kindly excuse me writing and asking some
> assistance from you as indeed I *very* much require it. . . .
> Two days ago I told you that the only notices the surgeons
> of our Hospital . . . had taken of acupressure was to send in
> a conjoint paper to the Managers making all surgical opera-
> tions to be stopped in my Ward No. 12—as well as in all the
> medical parts of the house, but my ward was specialised by
> name. Yesterday they (these surgeons) were asked to meet the
> Managers and explain their request. Mr Syme was spokes-
> man and indulged the Managers in all sorts of abuse against
> Dr Keiller and me. He was for having us at once prohibited
> from operating for vesico-vaginal fistulae, polypi etc. etc. in
> short for shutting up my ward. . . . I was not present while
> all this abuse was stated by Mr Syme and the attendant staff of
> surgeons. . . . My informant was one of the Managers who
> honestly states to me that they are so terrified of Syme that
> he will carry probably a majority of the Managers with
> him. . . .

Now is not all this persecution, for trying to do good in my profession, very hard. I would almost be ashamed to tell you how very, very hard indeed I feel it to be. . . . My friend among the Managers advised me to get a letter from any London surgeons to defend myself and my patients with. But as *here* the surgeons have *all* turned against me since my notices of acupressure I don't know in what direction really to turn. . . . I have not (to tell you the truth) heart and strength at present for such a fight.

Wells was asked to write a letter emphasising the importance of Simpson's previous work and how all the advances in surgery emanating from Edinburgh in the last 10 years had come from the obstetric department while there had been nothing from the surgeons. The letter continued: [166]

. . . if you only knew how heart sick and depressed I feel at these proceedings (which appears to *me* at least so much against all liberal feeling and against the whole spirit of the age we live) that I almost think you would excuse me troubling you with all these sorrows of mine. Till yesterday I fancied the Managers would not listen to Mr Syme's request; I am astonished certainly to hear they not only will listen but probably will act upon it unless I make some movement or another. My first impression was to give it all up and send in my resignation. But my duty to my Class and my poor patients is to make an attempt at the preservation of my rights.

His appeal was answered and Spencer Wells sent a letter in support. The proposal of the surgeons was defeated but the stage was set for a prolonged and bitter confrontation. In April 1860 Syme went to London to read a paper on the treatment of axillary aneurysm. In the discussion which followed he was asked what he thought about acupressure. He seized the opportunity to castigate Simpson, to decry the method and to suggest that no one would ever have taken notice of it had it not been published by the *Medical Times* which paper, he averred, was under Simpson's control! Spencer Wells rose to Simpson's defence and extolled acupressure as a technique which had a great future. The *Medical Times* then published a leader deploring that Syme should have criticised a brother professor in his absence. The writer, perhaps Spencer Wells, himself, stated 'Mr Syme has acquired considerable proficiency in the training of surgical adolescents, and he has some real merit as a practical surgeon' but rubbed in once more that it was to Simpson's labours that the Edinburgh School of Surgery owed its chief reputation. Simpson appreciated all this and he wrote to Wells: [167]

I cannot tell you how very grateful I feel for your kind defence of me at the Medico-Chirurgical Society. Surely the President ought not to have allowed any personal observations to be made against an absent member of the profession. . . . Some of Syme's greatest supporters here are wroth at him. It was (argued one of them to me two days ago) bringing 'the whole Edinburgh profession into discredit before their London brethren'. Is it not amusing to find acupressure . . . used in the Hospital at Naples and never once used in the Hospital at Edinburgh. His surgical colleagues are all afraid of our surgical 'Bomba'. It seems that I had mortally offended him by exposing his attempt, by the new Ordinances for Degrees at the University—to drive *all* students to attend *his* class.

There were, in fact, many other quarrels going on in Edinburgh, particularly concerning the medical curriculum on which Syme tended to express dictatorial opinions. Syme in attacking Simpson over acupressure was undoubtedly aiming to crush his influence completely.

It all became rather boring to the outside world. Interest in the new discovery in London was extinguished and the surgeons there sat back to watch what they now regarded as a childish and insignificant local slanging match. In a review of Simpson's book published in 1864 it had already been regretted 'that in Edinburgh what ought to be matters of scientific discussion merely have found a tendency to become subjects of personal squabbling . . .'. Simpson, rather wearily, carried on the fight, methodically collecting all the reports he could from the few surgeons who supported him and writing repeatedly to the journals with these collective results.

In Edinburgh the culmination of the whole affair was in a crisis early in 1865 and this perhaps marks the end of Simpson's fervent mission to popularise acupressure. When he published his book in 1864 there were some favourable reviews but others were highly critical. He replied to the critics with a pamphlet *Answers to the various objections against acupressure*. Syme had made some of the objections and had meanwhile advanced the counter-proposal that ligation of arteries might in some instances be replaced by the well tried method of torsion. In the preface to his pamphlet Simpson made special reference to the 'foolish' suggestions of Syme. Once more a single word triggered off a quarrel and this time Syme registered protest in a dramatic fashion which ensured the maximum of publicity. In front of his surgical class and some of his colleagues Syme tore up the offending publication. A correspondent described the episode for the *Edinburgh Daily Review*: [168]

> Strange scene in the University of Edinburgh: It is often stated that when the notorious surgical teacher Paracelsus, wished to show his aversion to any particular author, he immolated the writing he dissented from in the presence of his pupils. We were not aware that this mediaeval practice has ever been adopted in any of our Scottish Universities till last week when it was followed out in one of the class rooms of the University of Edinburgh. . . . Lately Dr Simpson issued a quiet pamphlet . . . Last week Mr Syme took this pamphlet into his classroom, and, without attempting to answer the rather unanswerable arguments which it contains in favour of acupressure, he scolded at the author and declared the pamphlet to be a piece of vulgar insolence. Then came the dénouement . . . With firm hand, teeth compressed, pale lines around his orbits and altogether a most determined and savage expression, he tore up the pamphlet with his fingers, and gave the fragments to his assistants to be consigned to the sawdust box with other surgical remains.

There were other versions of the scene given in the current medical journals. From there it is clear that the occasion was one of Syme's clinical lectures and the place was the operating theatre. Syme's action was almost certainly premeditated for he had invited some of his colleagues for the express purpose of witnessing his action. Dr John Brown was present and as he was then the assessor to the Chancellor of the University many deplored his presence in that it suggested official approbation of Syme's insolence.

The medical journals were on Simpson's side and attacked

Syme for behaviour which they considered unforgivable. The day after the episode the students crowded to Simpson's lecture room hoping for some equally vigorous reaction. They were disappointed for Simpson preserved his dignity and made little comment.

Syme was not one to tolerate criticism in the medical journals or anywhere else. He at once wrote to justify his action. He indicated that he had seen it as his duty to express publicly his complete disapproval of acupressure and that he had felt it necessary to reply to a personal affront by a personal attack. Simpson could no longer remain silent and sent long letters to the medical press. He recalled Syme's attack on him in London five years before. He justified answering Syme's criticisms of acupressure just as he had felt it necessary to reply to the criticisms of others. He empha- sised that Syme had never even tried acupressure and that his chief objection to it was that it had been invented by an obstetrician. Finally he considered that Syme, as a member of the General Medical Council, had in his behaviour shown a very bad example to his students. These letters were very reasonable and there were many who felt that Syme should apologise to end the matter. Syme had no intention of apologising and the correspondence ground on for another year with mutual abuse and recrimination. Syme finally with- drew from the correspondence and dismissed the whole affair by writing: [169]

> Your obstetric correspondent can hardly expect that after the public execution of his obnoxious pamphlet any amount of personal abuse or professional misrepresentation proceeding from him should be decreed worthy of my notice.

This was Syme's usual way of ending a public argument and it left the opponent furious but impotent. The major issue of the merits or demerits of acupressure was lost in these trivial exchanges at a personal level. Syme by his calculated act to publicise his antagonism to acupressure had in fact achieved his purpose. By 1867 acupressure was used by few surgeons and forgotten by most. Already the problems which Simpson had striven to solve were being overcome by another, Joseph Lister. There was cruel irony for Simpson in the fact that Lister was the protégé of Syme and the failure to gain acceptance of acupressure must have been all the harder for Simpson to bear for this reason.

It is easy to dismiss acupressure as of minor importance in the history of surgery. Today the word is almost forgotten or is vaguely confused with acupuncture. A few medical historians make a passing reference to Simpson's 'skewers', tolerantly regarding his work as a rather eccentric excursion into a field which did not really concern him and recalling with some relish Syme's 'execution' of the pamphlet. It may be wrong to accept this assessment and it is a scant tribute to Simpson to dismiss in this way a work to which he gave so much of his life.

Without the advantage of knowledge of Pasteur's work on fermentation and bacterial action (a knowledge available to Lister and the basis of all his work) Simpson by intuition, observation and experiment established some very simple and important facts. It can be accepted with some confidence that much of the wound infection in the pre-antiseptic period was due to the effects of the combination of septic ligature material and dead tissue. Acupressure was thus an ingenious and logical means of diminishing wound infection. There were, of course, snags about the technique and Simpson himself admitted how difficult it was to describe it in writing. Unfortunately he never seemed to have had the assistance of an artist who could produce the three-dimensional drawings which were essential to the readers' understanding. The placing of the needles was exceedingly tricky and few surgeons took the trouble to use them exactly as Simpson described. To most the method seemed precarious in the extreme. It must surprise any modern surgeon that it was possible to control a large artery such as the femoral by the external pressure of a needle held in place only by fixation to the adjacent soft tissues. Nevertheless there were some surgeons who achieved this and they were rewarded by a much higher rate of primary healing than could have been expected from the old methods. That Lister's successful introduction of the sterile catgut ligature eliminated in one stroke the necessity for acupressure does not devaluate Simpson's work. Simpson himself perhaps overestimated the importance of his discovery and to some extent, like most inventors, may have become rather obsessed with its merits. He always said, however, that he hoped that one day something better would be devised. He must be given full credit for the principles he taught.[170]

The merit of his work must be assessed more fully than in a simple evaluation of the technique which he proposed. Attention has already been drawn to the wide scope of his book in which inevitably there is much space devoted to the actual method and to the results. There are chapters, however, which can be read with advantage today, for although Simpson was not primarily a surgeon he grasped the principles of surgical technique surprisingly well. Apart from his exposure of the perils of burying septic ligatures he propounded sound ideas about wound closure and dressings. He stressed the necessity of careful apposition of wounds without tension, of closing dead spaces, of irrigating wounds to remove all dead or foreign tissue before attempting closure, of achieving complete haemastasis, of providing dependent drainage when necessary and of absolute rest for a wound. 'All touching and fingering of the sides or vicinities of recent wounds should be avoided and forbidden' was one of his aphorisms (a warning which was very pertinent at the time). He scorned the use of multiple dressings and packs but advocated that wounds should be left exposed to the air to let nature do the healing. Such principles were steps towards aseptic surgery and remain as important today as ever. In this advice, supported by a mass of clinical observations and experiments, Simpson presented an exposition of technique which surpassed any in the standard surgical text books of the day.

He sent a copy of his book to Lister in 1865 (Lister was then Professor of Surgery in Glasgow): [171]

I have taken the liberty of sending you a book on acupressure: and I hope you will do me the favour of kindly accepting it.

Of its size I am quite ashamed: but it spun out to an extent I had no dream of when I began.

I am sanguine enough to have no fears whatever of the ultimate adoption of acupressure or some similar haemostatic. But a long stretch of time is required for all such chances. Yet in 50 months it has progressed more, I believe, than the ligature did in its first 50 years. To my 'medical' mind it

appears most strange and inexplicable that surgeons do go on
sedulously and systematically implanting by the ligature two,
four, six or more fragments of *dead* flesh and decomposing
arterial tissue in every large wound: and yet say they wish
these wounds to heal by the first intention. When the very
practice of thus placing dead fragments between the lips of
wounds, is, among the least, to prevent adhesions succeeding.
It is the stranger when all late experience has proved that the
needle is, *at least, as* effective a haemostatic as the ligature.

But all this apparent paradox is merely perhaps from my
taking a medical view of a surgical subject. . . .

Lister, with his astute and critical mind, must already have
studied Simpson's arguments and understood them better
than most surgeons. Although there is evidence that Lister
had little faith in acupressure as a method of controlling
bleeding vessels, Simpson's ideas may well have stimulated
the subsequent evolution of the antiseptic method by the
younger man. The controversy on acupressure must have
done much to pave the way for the ultimate acceptance of
Lister's ideas, in that it induced in the minds of surgeons
a more critical attitude towards the problem of wound infection. Acupressure can, therefore, be legitimately seen as a
significant contribution towards the conquest of this the
greatest hazard of surgery. Lister may have placed the key-
stone on the arch of the edifice but Simpson certainly
strengthened the foundations.

The second surgical controversy concerned ovariotomy.
This is of considerable historical importance because it was
the experience of the ovariotomists which led in time to the
full development of abdominal surgery. When Syme and
Simpson started their careers abdominal abscesses were
drained, hernias were repaired and occasionally an operation
was done for tumour or obstruction. In general, however,
there was a great reluctance to explore the abdominal cavity
and this persisted even after general anaesthesia was introduced. This was in part because of a fear that the entry of
air would inevitably prove fatal. Sepsis, then unexplained,
was as great a risk in an abdominal operation as in any other
so-called capital procedures such as major amputations, but
this risk did not deter the surgeon from a heroic amputation.

The pathologists knew much about abdominal diseases and, in particular, of the ovarian cyst or 'encysted dropsy of the ovary'. They recognised this as a tumour which could be diagnosed fairly accurately and which grew slowly but inexorably to a very large size. It was known that the victim in time suffered great discomfort and that she might become emaciated and die. Usually the tumour was mobile and attached only by a local stalk or pedicle of blood vessels and so to some bolder surgeons it seemed logical to advocate operative removal and to expect that control of the cut pedicle would offer no great technical difficulty. Few were prepared to defy convention and make the attempt.

There are many full accounts of the history of ovariotomy and here it is sufficient to highlight the events having some association with Edinburgh. A break-through came in 1809 when Ephraim McDowell (1771–1830), a country surgeon of Kentucky, removed such a cyst with recovery of the patient. He published this case with three other successes in 1817. He had studied for a while in Edinburgh under John Bell and dutifully sent a copy of his paper to his former teacher. Bell had retired to Italy for his health and the report was read by his assistant John Lizars. Almost certainly encouraged by McDowell's success Lizars, in the short space of four months, did four abdominal operations; in each with the intention of removing a cyst. His technique was crude and considering that it is reported that at one operation every spectator in turn put his hand into the abdomen it is surprising that three of the four patients survived. In only one case was a cyst removed successfully but this was a remark-achievement. Lizars quite rightly felt that he had demonstrated the feasibility of removing an ovarian cyst and he forecast that other abdominal conditions might justifiably be treated by operation. When he published his results in 1825 he was attacked fiercely and unfairly by all his colleagues, particularly Liston who described him as a 'belly ripper'. Opinion was so overwhelmingly against Lizars that he never again attempted another abdominal operation of this type. Even today there is reluctance to credit Lizars with success but a study of his detailed case reports and plates is absolutely convincing. He unquestionably earns a place in history as the first to remove an ovarian cyst in Great Britain. For the next 20 years, despite the gradual accumulation of a few successes elsewhere, no one in Edinburgh dared to repeat the performance.[172]

In 1842 Charles Clay of Manchester, an Edinburgh graduate who had been present at Lizars' operations, began a long series of ovariotomies. Despite vehement criticism he achieved in the next 15 years more successes than those totalled by all other surgeons in Great Britain. Clay corresponded with Simpson and kept him up to date with his results. Right from the start Simpson was prepared to look at Clay's work without bias, unlike his more bigoted surgical colleagues. In September 1845 ovariotomy was once more attempted in Edinburgh. A woman of 20 was admitted to the Infirmary under the care of the physician Dr Hughes Bennet. Syme had already tapped the cyst and drawn off five gallons of fluid; this was the treatment employed by most surgeons. The patient remained ill despite the reduction in size of the cyst and Simpson was called to give a further opinion. At his suggestion more fluid was taken off but still she worsened. Dr Bennet 'proposed to the acting surgeons severally the operation of ovariotomy, which they declined to perform'. The distressed woman was discharged to her lodgings there to continue under the care of Peter Handyside (1808–1881), a young surgeon and a well known teacher of anatomy. There was a consultation between Handyside, Bennet and Simpson and at last it was agreed that an operation should be attempted. Next day this was done by Handyside in the presence of Simpson, Bennet, Goodsir and several other doctors. Syme, who most likely was one of the surgeons who earlier had advised against operation, was not present. The abdomen was opened and the cyst partially extracted. Simpson supported the tumour and Goodsir pressed down the sides of the wound to keep the intestines from escaping. A huge cyst on the left ovary was then removed by dividing its pedicle. The vessels were secured with silk and the long ends of the ligature were brought out through the wound in the accepted manner. She did well at first and seemed to be recovering but on the 70th post-operative day she died. An autopsy revealed obstruction of the intestine from adhesions and there were other complications of sepsis.[173, 174]

The operation was done on the lines proposed by Clay and aroused great interest and much criticism when it was reported to the Medico-Chirurgical Society early in 1845. Bennet and Handyside defended the propriety of operating in similar progressive cases, despite the fatal issue. The meeting was adjourned so that there could be a fuller discussion. Dr Cormack then condemned the operation completely. Simpson supported Handyside but stressed the difficulties of management when an obstetrician made the diagnosis and a surgeon was called to do the operation. 'Surgeons,' he said, 'as a class still confessedly allow themselves to be swayed by the trammels of authority, and the mere fact that some of the highest names in surgery had once declared (with or without due investigation) against ovariotomy, is with most others an ample and satisfactory reason for rejecting the operation.' From the available statistics he showed that ovariotomy was no more dangerous than a major amputation and he quoted Clay's remarkable success. He forecast improvements in the technique of handling the vascular pedicle of the tumour and gave a fair review of the whole situation. Mr Spence rose to the defence of the surgeons but was unconvincing in his arguments against Simpson's better informed comments. Syme was not present and the editor of the journal in which the discussion was recorded regretted that more of the teachers of surgery or surgeons to the Infirmary, excepting Handyside and Spence, had not favoured the Society with their opinions.

The attitude of the Edinburgh surgeons in 1845 was the same as that of the London surgeons. It remained for Simpson to go on publicising the good results achieved by Clay and to encourage others to do the operation. He may, about this date, have attempted it himself. There is some doubt about this for in none of his writings does he ever give a clear record of his own experience of ovariotomy. During a discussion in July 1847 on ether anaesthesia Syme attacked Simpson for his advocacy of ovariotomy and alleged that there had been three such operations 'performed by the Professor of Midwifery or under his auspices, the whole of which had proved fatal'. Simpson did not deny this. In the numerous reviews of reported cases of ovariotomy up to 1848 Simpson's name appears only once; he had apparently communicated verbally 'a fatal case that occurred to himself, the only instance he has operated'. Simpson brought Clay up to Edinburgh in March 1848 to give a lecture. He said that although they could give chloroform in Edinburgh they could not do ovariotomies, while it was the reverse in Manchester! He then demonstrated his skill (his twenty-eighth ovariotomy) but, regrettably, the patient died the next day.[175]

In 1850 ovariotomy was denounced so effectively in London by Dr Lee, supported by most of the better known surgeons of the teaching hospitals, that no one there dared to do it. Charles Clay, almost alone in England, carried on the fight. Unfortunately he did not inspire confidence, partly because he was a mere provincial and partly because he was careless with his statistics.

The next publicised operation in Edinburgh was not until October 1856. Once more Simpson was involved. The surgeon was A. M. Edwards (?–1868); Simpson induced anaesthesia with chloroform and then moved round to help to lift the tumour out of the abdomen. The patient died of a chest complication five days later. The case was duly reported and once more there was a full discussion at the Medico-Chirurgical Society. Matthews Duncan was against the operation and Simpson put the case in favour of it. He quoted Clay's now remarkable series of 71 patients of which 49 had recovered. The discussion ended with Professor Miller, the President of the Society, giving a cautious summing-up which indicated that few were on Simpson's side.[176]

Late in 1857, in London, Spencer Wells attacked the problem afresh and by 1865 he convinced even the most sceptical that ovariotomy was relatively safe and a justifiable procedure. Wells was in close touch with Simpson all this time and kept him informed of his results. In June 1859 he wrote to Simpson: [177]

I did another ovariotomy three weeks ago—the patient is convalescent. I do another tomorrow and one next week. So far my success has been four out of five—But I suppose one can hardly expect to continue in that proportion.

Wells' cautious optimism was justified and his success

continued. He achieved this because he adopted a method of control of the ovarian pedicle which ensured that if the stump became infected there was little risk of abscess or peritonitis. He brought the stump outside the wall of the abdomen and held it there for several days by a special clamp which was detached when healing had progressed. In doing this he was preaching the same lesson as Simpson in his advocacy of acupressure, that surgeons should not leave dead tissue in contact with a long septic ligature in the depths of a wound or in a body cavity. The method was clumsy but safer than any other at the time. When in 1868 Lister introduced the sterile catgut ligature and the additional protection against infection provided by his antiseptic methods, Wells was able to discard the clamp. Before 1868 Wells had shown that it was possible to do abdominal operations with reasonable safety. Simpson was intensely interested in Wells' success and on more than one occasion went to London to see him operate. He tried to persuade Wells to occlude the pedicle by fixing it to the under surface of the abdominal wall with a large acupressure needle. In an undated letter Simpson writes: [178]

> I am sadly and powerfully tempted to run up and see your ovariotomy tomorrow: but I cannot well escape for a day at present. In the first dissection that occurs, please try the acupressure of the stalk on the dead body, you will see that you can perfectly command it on the living.

This seems to have been rather a precarious technique to suggest and Wells did not try it. Simpson, however, used a modified acupressure to control the pedicle in at least one case.

In his many papers on diseases of the ovary Simpson repeatedly stressed the limitations of treatment of cysts by tapping and pressed for the readier acceptance of operative removal. In 1863, in reporting an operation he himself had done successfully, he deplored the continued opposition of the surgeon but hinted that even Syme was beginning to give rather cautious approval. A letter from Christison to Dr Dewar in February 1863 is informative. Dewar had sought advice concerning his wife who had an ovarian tumour: [179]

> I saw Syme on the morning after I called on you. He advised me

strongly to see, in preference to any one else, Dr T. Keith. . . .

Syme, as usual, is very clear in his views. He was for long opposed to the operation on three grounds, because the diagnosis of ovarian tumour was then uncertain, because the prognosis in cases of operation was very unfavourable and because the proper mode of operating was ill-ascertained. But now he admits ovarian excision into the category of allowable operations. . . . He will not himself perform it. But he has nothing now to object to its performance by others. It is best, he thinks, to leave it in the hands of obstetrical practitioners. . . .

Dr T. Keith assents to all Mr Syme's doctrine. . . . He has done it thrice. Twice it has proved successful. . . .

Syme had been converted but it is curious that he should have favoured the performance of the operation by the obstetrician, for he was always very much against obstetricians doing any surgery outside their immediate province. Perhaps he really felt that as long as the obstetrician was not Simpson all would be well! It is surprising too that Syme himself was not prepared to undertake this kind of surgery for he had never lacked boldness. He did not seem to see in the rising success of ovariotomy a challenge to the surgeon and almost limitless possibilities in the management of diseases of other abdominal organs.

The reference in the letter to Keith is significant. Thomas Keith had, like his brother George, been apprenticed to Simpson and trained by him in obstetrics and gynaecology. Simpson encouraged him to take up ovariotomy and sent him to London to see Wells operate. By 1870 Keith completed 100 ovariotomies with only 17 deaths, figures which surpassed even those of Wells. Much of his success was due to the fact that he, like Wells, operated in a small private hospital and that his patients thus escaped contact with the infection so rife in the general wards of any large hospital. He received the appointment of 'extra-surgeon for ovariotomy' to the Royal Infirmary and was accepted as the expert in Edinburgh. He ranks with Wells as a great pioneer in abdominal surgery. Syme referred most of his cases of ovarian tumour to Keith. Simpson did likewise until early in 1867 when he wrote to Keith concerning a patient:[180]

The bearer was sent down to me to have ovariotomy performed. As I do not feel strong enough for additional work
and anxiety and possibly may be off to Paris when the session
closes this week I have sent her in to be under your care and
to operate if you think the case a proper one.

To Simpson's dismay Keith refused the case and there
followed a miserable and prolonged correspondence. Keith
accused Simpson of having 'spoken against him professionally'. Some years previously after seeing a similar patient in
consultation with Simpson, Keith had operated without asking his senior to be present. No doubt Simpson had at the
time expressed his disapproval of this breach of etiquette but
there may have been other reasons for a quarrel. It was in
great sorrow that Simpson wrote to Keith: [181]

Weigh in your own heart and conscience whether your conduct
be truly that of a professional gentleman and a professsed
Christian. I am indeed sorry that the sons of your honoured
father should so behave. . . . Without my assistance, in the
first instance, whence would have been derived the practice
which you now enjoy. . . . I think life is far too brief and
too precious for perpetuating such miserable misunderstandings as those betwixt you and me and I was desirous and I
still truly am, to end them.

The olive branch was not accepted and Keith severed his
connection and his friendship with his teacher. There was a
final snub: [182]

. . . in regard to ovariotomy at least we had better follow each
our own road. That our surgical ideas and our notions (as to
what is right and proper for those who commit their lives
to our skill and care) are entirely at variance cannot be better
indicated than by you having ventured to do no less than
three ovarian operations at one sitting—a proceeding which
to me is simply incomprehensible.

It must be admitted that Simpson's own success as an ovariotomist was very limited. It is apparent that he did not record
his failures. Whether or not he attempted what would have
been the exceptional performance of polishing off three
ovariotomies in an afternoon, as Keith so deplored, is unknown. Even Spencer Wells in his prime was content to con-

centrate on one case a day and rarely did two! However this may be Simpson must be given credit for appreciating at an early stage that ovariotomy offered great possibilities and for encouraging its more general adoption. It is probable that his support of Spencer Wells assisted the latter to overcome the opposition which he encountered in London.

Syme took a much longer time to give even a limited approval to the operation. He was heavily prejudiced for many reasons and perhaps most of all because it was Lizars who had made the first attempt in Edinburgh. In his address on surgery at the annual meeting of the British Medical Association in Leamington, Syme once more attacked Lizars: [183]

> We now come to ovariotomy which has of late been the subject of so much attention; and it will here, perhaps, be supposed that a claim for the honour of priority may be advanced on the part of Edinburgh, where the operation was first performed. But to confess the truth I fear the northern metropolis, so far from deserving any credit on this account, should rather plead guilty to having invested the procedure with an aspect so repulsive as to impede rather than promote its adoption. It was brought forward by the same person who had proposed to remedy hypertrophy of the heart by blowing air into the pericardium, to puncture the brain in acute hydrocephalus and to treat enlargement of the prostate by cutting out the entire gland: so that the profession in Edinburgh were not either disposed to adopt the excision of ovarian tumours, or at all surprised by the results of its attempted performance.

He then went on to misrepresent Lizars' cases completely and to blame him entirely for the failure of Edinburgh surgeons to contribute to the solution of the problems of ovariotomy in the early days. He had to admit the success of Spencer Wells and he did pay tribute to Thomas Keith, claiming him as his protégé. He forgot the primitive circumstances in which Lizars had operated in 1825. Syme had accepted the unjust condemnations by Liston and other surgeons. In this denunciation five years after Lizars' death Syme was shown in a most unforgiving character.

From about 1864 onwards Syme collaborated closely with Keith and was present when he did some of his earlier ovariotomies. Lister was present at Keith's eleventh case and assisted George Buchanan of Glasgow in 1862 with an un-successful attempt. Lister, however, inherited some of Syme's attitudes towards abdominal operations in that he likewise never attempted ovariotomy, even with the protection of anti-septics. Lister was nevertheless intensely interested in the application of his principles to abdominal surgery and did follow closely the rapid developments which took place after ovariotomy was established.

The last ovariotomy in which Simpson was involved was an unfortunate case. Already tired and ill he went in January 1870 to Alloa to assist his friend Dr Brotherstone. Simpson gave the anaesthetic and before Brotherstone had opened the abdomen the patient died. It was a typical chloroform death and was widely publicised. One of Simpson's last com-munications to the medical press was to maintain that this was a chance death due to the operation and nothing to do with chloroform. It was a sad climax to all Simpson had done to advance the cause of the ovariotomists. That his influence was much greater than that of Syme is unquestionable. It is noteworthy that when Professor Courty of Montpellier pub-lished an account of a visit to Great Britain in 1864 he dedicated his book to Simpson for his part in establishing ovariotomy.[184, 185]

CHAPTER 10

Listerism and Hospitalism

THE introduction in 1867 by Joseph Lister of the anti-septic system was one of the greatest advances in medical science in the nineteenth century. Lister's work cannot be looked at in isolation but 'came as the culmination of several decades of hypothesis and experiment which were tending in the direction which he followed'. The slowness with which his teaching was accepted, particularly by the surgeons, is explained in part by the fact that 'he was preaching to a profession largely untrained in science'. It must be recorded, however, that Lister, despite his single-minded devotion to his task, was surprisingly ill-informed of much that had been written which had relevance to the problems he sought to solve. He had, for example, to admit that when in 1865 he first applied antiseptic principles in the treatment of compound fractures he had not heard of the significant work of Semmelweis. There were others such as Gordon of Aberdeen, White of Manchester and the American Oliver Wendell Holmes who had already taught, as Semmelweis demonstrated so dramatically, that infection in childbirth was often transmitted from one patient to another by the hands, clothing or instruments of the attendant. A direct contagion, so well recognised in the propagation of puerperal fever, was long ignored by the surgeons mainly because of their failure to equate 'surgical fever' and 'puerperal fever'. It is perhaps to Lister's credit that without being fully aware of principles established so clearly by some obstetricians he evolved his own theory so successfully. It may even be that his scientific approach was aided because he was untram-melled by a mass of ill-proven or ill-supported doctrines. Lister's work must be seen against contemporary scientific

196

beliefs, in particular the conception of spontaneous generation of living forms. To the average doctor, whatever his
specialty, the interpretation of current scientific view points
offered great difficulty and confusion. While the use of the
essential tool, the microscope, had developed rapidly, the
techniques of staining and isolation of organisms were crude.
Although the existence of simple cellular forms of life had
long been recognised, their morphology and behaviour was
often fitted to pre-conceived theory. Lister had the advantage
of having inherited from his father an interest and skill in the
use of the microscope and this expertise ensured that his
interpretation of the pathology of inflammation was sound
and profitable. He was unique amongst surgeons in his ability
to apply to a clinical problem a truly scientific method of
elucidation.

His contemporaries, with few exceptions, had acquired
from their stereotyped training far less ability and enthusiasm
to use the new weapons such as the microscope and far less
readiness to question established dogma. Simpson was one
exception, as he showed so constantly in all his career. From
his earliest years he saw in the problems of wound infection
a great challenge; this he accepted and although he sometimes took the wrong path his contributions were of great
significance. Syme had a less direct influence in these events,
and some have said that his only contribution was his happy
choice of Lister as his assistant, but this is an understatement.
A review of the parts played by the two men in the prolonged
struggle against hospital infection, in all its wide context, is
relevant not only to accord appropriate credit but also to
bring out further aspects of their characters. Both lived to see
the end of the beginning of the conquest of a major scourge
of mankind. Inevitably there was a personal conflict but
perhaps this brought some advantage in that it made others
think and may have done something to clear the air for the
eventual acceptance of Lister's doctrines.

It has been told how Simpson, by his introduction of acupressure, believed he could eliminate particular factors in
wound infection. This was a specialised approach and he
knew well that it could deal with only a part of the problem.
He viewed hospital infection from a much wider angle. An

interest in epidemiology was first shown when, about 1838, he wrote a pamphlet *On the evidence of the occasional propagation of malignant cholera*. In this he discussed the accepted views on the transmission of the disease, then sweeping Europe in repeated epidemics. He came down on the side of those who believed that there was often a direct contagion from one victim to another. The evidence he presented was largely from his brief experience as a general practitioner in Bathgate. It was his obstetrical experience which stimulated him further, for soon he saw confirmation of the contagious nature of puerperal fever. He was quicker than most to suspect, and then accept, that puerperal and surgical fever were analagous and that the lessons which were so clear to some obstetricians should be digested by the surgeons. There is a strong hint that as early as 1840 he recommended that surgeons should take more care to cleanse their instruments so that they would avoid the transfer of 'morbific' material from one patient to the other. In 1851 he stated that for many years he had used a solution of cyanide of potassium to wash his hands before operating and so it may be that he used this effective measure before it was proved to be essential by Semmelweis in 1847.

Ignaz Semmelweis (1815–1865) working in Vienna in 1846, observed that in the lying-in wards attended by medical students there was a mortality from puerperal sepsis three times greater than that in the wards attended only by midwives. The death of a friend from septicaemia after a wound inflicted while doing an autopsy convinced him that puerperal and surgical fever were similar. It was significant that in Vienna the students were taught obstetrics on the eviscerated bodies of women who had died in child birth, almost invariably of infection. He made his students cleanse their hands with chlorinated water when they came from the deadhouse to the lying-in wards. The result was dramatic, as the mortality rate in the students' wards at once fell to that in the midwives' wards. Although his observations were attacked vehemently by his senior colleagues he convinced some of his pupils, including visitors from other countries, that he was right. He himself was reluctant to publish these findings and only a short account was printed by his colleague Hebra in

December 1847. It was not until 1861 that Semmelweis wrote a full account of his work. In his lifetime he was given little credit and no reward for his outstanding discovery and he died in 1865 disillusioned and insane.[186]

A few surgeons from England visited Vienna about 1846 and saw the effects of his teaching, for Vienna was then a centre of instruction for the aspiring surgeon or obstetrician. Amongst them was Charles Routh (1822–1909), a young London doctor, who was later to be associated with the Samaritan Hospital where Wells did most of his pioneer work in ovariotomy. When Routh came home he read a paper, in 1848, to the Medico-Chirurgical Society of London and he gave a clear account of Semmelweis's work with statistics which should have convinced his audience. In the discussion which followed it was clear that few were impressed. Simpson may have read this paper and, in addition, there is the suggestion that he had a letter from Dr Arneth of Vienna. It is said that Simpson was not initially in agreement with Semmelweis's theories but this was perhaps due to a misunderstanding of the use of the term contagion. In 1850, probably on Simpson's invitation, Arneth came to Edinburgh and he described in a lecture the astonishing success which had followed the simple precautions introduced in Vienna. There was a lively discussion in which Simpson now paid a generous tribute to Semmelweis. It is likely that when Spencer Wells visited Vienna in 1848 on a prolonged continental study tour he learnt of Semmelweis's doctrines. Certainly when Wells started to do ovariotomies he insisted that all spectators should sign a statement that in the previous week they had not been present at an autopsy or dealt with a septic case.[187]

Simpson's views on hospital infection had begun to take a positive shape by 1849 when he read to the Obstetrical Society a report on the work of the Edinburgh Royal Maternity Hospital. His statistics were significant for he had found that one out of 53 women delivered in hospital had died compared with one out of 270 delivered at home. In the majority of fatal cases death was from some variant of sepsis. He stated his conclusions boldly: [188]

Everyone acquainted with hospital practice, whether obstetric, surgical or medical, is well aware of the great liability among the patients to febrile and inflammatory attacks whenever the wards are overcrowded: and in no practice is this more visible than in midwifery. Indeed I believe that there are few or no circumstances which would contribute more to save surgical and obstetric patients from phlebitic and other analogous disorders, than a total change in the present system of hospital practice. I have often stated and taught, that if our present medical surgical and obstetric hospitals were changed from being crowded palaces, with a layer of sick in each flat, into villages or cottages, with one or at most two patients in each room, a great saving of life would be effected. And if the village were constructed of iron (as is now sometimes done for other purposes), instead of brick or stone, it could be taken down and rebuilt every few years; a matter apparently of much moment in hospital hygiene. Besides the value of the material would not greatly deteriorate from use; the principal outlay would be the first cost of it. It could be erected in any vacant space or spaces of ground, within or around a city, that chanced to be unoccupied; and, in cases of epidemics, the accommodation could always be at once and readily increased.

This was his first public utterance on a subject which later was to be termed 'hospitalism', the concept that infection was largely related to the faulty design, ventilation and management of large hospitals. For the rest of his life Simpson toiled to convert his colleagues to these beliefs and when he died he was still firmly convinced that he was right. In countless papers he expanded these ideas and he collected a mass of figures to prove his points. Most of his teaching was based on sound arguments and must be viewed in relation to the dreadful conditions in hospitals at this time.

In 1850 there was another important paper, *On the Analogy between Puerperal Fever and Surgical Fever*. He had, of course, long accepted this analogy: [189]

. . . observing (what I have taught for the last ten years) that there exists, I believe, on record, a series of facts amply sufficient to prove that patients during labour have been inoculated with a materia morbi capable of enciting puerperal fever and this materia morbi is liable to be inoculated by the fingers of the attendant.

The mode of infection in puerperal fever needed reemphasis for despite all that had been recorded previously many had forgotten its importance. To some of the more fashionable accoucheurs it was a terrible insult that anyone should suggest that they were the carriers of disease. In this paper Simpson went on to insist once more that the preventitive methods known to the obstetricians should be applied to surgical practice. The close relationship between surgical fever and puerperal fever was still consistently denied by many and was still argued about as late as 1875. There was a degree of mysticism over the disorders which followed childbirth and fashionable but vague theories were discarded with reluctance. Simpson made his case from careful analysis and comparison of the accepted local and general effects on the two conditions and proved the analogy with absolute clarity. There was for him, as for most doctors at this date, a crucial gap in understanding, the acceptance of the germ theory of disease. This seems to have eluded Simpson almost to his dying day but he did accept that infection was due to a contagious material which he thought to be akin to the inoculable matter of small-pox. This was a logical theory and a great advance on the current obscure ideas of putrefaction, decomposition of tissue by oxidation and the mysterious influence of the atmosphere known as miasma.

In summary it may be said that he elaborated on three principles. Firstly he insisted that by applying the lessons learned in obstetrics surgeons could go far towards controlling the incidence of wound infection. Secondly he believed that by altering hospital design the environment of the patient would be so changed that the risks of sepsis would be greatly diminished. Thirdly in acupressure he was convinced that he had introduced an operative technique which would go far towards eliminating wound infection. These three beliefs were complementary and it is astonishing that they were worked out so effectively by one man.

A published lecture, *Surgical Fevers*, in 1859 expresses Simpson's opinions in their entirety and the quotations which follow are in answer to the question, 'What do patients die of after undergoing surgical operations, either in the course of general or obstetric surgery?': [190]

There is not a text-book of midwifery in which there is not

one lengthy chapter devoted to puerperal fever, the common cause of death in obstetrical patients . . . there is hardly a large work in surgery in which you will find a word stated as to the cause of mortality of patients who have been subjected to surgical operations.

Faithful to their designations and their original vocation, surgeons have, with some great and brilliant exceptions, gone on trying to improve the merely manual part of their profession—what some have spoken of as the cutlery and carpentry of surgery only, without attending sufficiently to some of its most important pathological relations. . . .

Indeed some surgeons seem to lose all interest in their patients from the time they are carried off the operating table, and eschew rather than otherwise their treatment, if they are attacked with surgical fever. . . .

We have seen that every patient who is placed upon an operation table runs no small risk of death and that, when operation is severe, the patient is in as great, or indeed greater danger than the soldier entering one of the bloodiest and most fatal battlefields.

He went on to define surgical fever as a constitutional disease accompanied by the development of local acute inflammation confined often to organs and tissues lying in the vicinity of the site of the wound or operation but in many cases diffused over other and more remote organs and tissues. While he regarded previous chronic disease of the liver, kidneys or spleen as predisposing to the disease, he again insisted on the vital factor as a morbid material which entered the wound. He demolished the theory that the disease was due to pus cells being absorbed into the circulation, citing many conditions in which the white cells in the blood increased in number without there being a primary source of pus. In prevention he insisted on the early operation, as for example in situations requiring amputation, a lesson fully learned in the Crimean War. Once more he argued against the use of large hospitals and emphasised the dangers of transmission of infection by surgeons and nurses. In the treatment of a wound he advocated careful closure, the avoidance of ligatures and the alternative of acupressure. There is a paragraph with a forecast of Lister's methods: [191]

In relation to the prophylaxis of surgical fever, the question is whether acid, chlorinated or other antiseptic applications employed in the first days or hours of primary wounds, would not in some cases and under some circumstances neutralise or destroy any septic poisons in these wounds.

For the constitutional effects of the surgical fever he favoured an empirical use of quinine, if the fever was intermittent in type. Unlike so many others he had no illusions about opium as a specific remedy but he recommended its use for the comfort of the patient. He favoured wine and brandy as stimulants and advised 'depuration' by sweating and by stimulating kidney function.

Simpson's criticism of the surgeons was justified. Although they knew that operations were often fatal and that the majority of deaths were caused by the complications of 'inflammation', whether local or general, few seemed to question the inevitability of it all. In the publication of successful operations, however, they were always relieved to record that after the operation there were 'no bad effects'. In the popular contemporary text-books of surgery, as for example the fifth edition of *A System of Practical Surgery* by William Fergusson published as late as 1870, we find 'pyaemia', 'erysipelas', 'hospital gangrene' and such fatal consequences of operative surgery described fully insofar as symptomology and treatment are concerned, but without the slightest reference to a possible cause or to their prevention. There is scarcely a hint that so large a proportion of patients died after operations. Thomas Holmes edited an elaborate *System of Surgery* in 1860 and from this too one may appreciate contemporary surgical views. Of the contributors John Simon writes on 'Inflammation'. The causes are listed variously as 'chemical violence', 'morbid production of the body itself', 'altered state of local nerves' and 'abnormal properties of circulatory blood'. Contagion is dismissed with the brief observations that vaccinia and syphilis may be inoculated by a septic lancet from person to person. It is thought possible that a few conditions other than such specific infections are contagious, but the only example given is infective ophthalmia while nothing is said of puerperal infection. Much is made of 'predisposition' to inflammation from 'molecular weakness of texture', malnutrition, alcoholism or intercurrent disease. He has little to suggest about treatment except for the usual empirical remedies, while 'antiseptics' are chosen for their deodorant properties. Campbell de Morgan, another London surgeon, was a little more original in his chapter on 'erysipelas', for he recognised the danger of using the same 'stinking' sponge on one patient's wound and then on another. He accepted that puerperal fever was an 'internal manifestation' of erysipelas but there is no suggestion for prevention. George Callender dealt with 'pyaemia' and dismisses the question of aetiology with the casual sentence: 'It signifies little whence these matters are derived, whether from decomposing pus, unhealthy secretions, decomposing hides, dead bodies, vegetable putrefactions or from animals suffering from acrid discharges.' Even James Paget, the most astute of the surgeon pathologists, could write in the section on wound healing without any discussion of the causes of failure. There is a chapter on 'Animal Poisons' in which Alfred Poland discusses 'dissection wounds'. Many a promising young surgeon died from an accidental wound incurred at operation or autopsy and this was the tragedy which put Semmelweis on the right track. Poland, and some other surgeons, although they recognised that some 'putrescent fluid' or 'specific virus' was inoculated, could not see the implications of such accidents.[192]

The inability or reluctance of surgeons to change their conceptions of inflammation is brought out by the fact that Fergusson, as acknowledged leader, even in 1870 dismissed Lister's work in a few lines without comment. From this it is all too clear that he had no understanding of the causes and no apparent interest in the prevention of infection in surgical operations:[193]

> Within these few years the use of carbolic acid in solution or in paste, has been extolled by Professor Lister, for cases of compound fracture, both as a deodorizer, and as having special virtues in preventing or limiting the formation of pus.

It cannot be said that Syme revealed in his lectures or his writings a positive and urgent approach to the problem of reducing the high mortality which followed surgical operations. Such efforts as he made in this direction were confined to the elaboration of the details of dressing wounds and he had strong views on this subject. The broader issues for long escaped him and he, like most of his London colleagues, accepted the extension of inflammation as a regrettable fact and scarcely questioned established theories.

At times, however, the conditions of his wards alarmed him. In 1843 there was an angry minute recorded by the Managers of the Royal Infirmary deploring that a woman who was badly burned had, on the instruction of the 'professors', been refused admission by the house-surgeon on the grounds that such cases 'stank all the wards and annoyed other patients'. Syme saw the document and took it as a censure on his conduct. He told the Managers that the hospital was in a 'frightfully unhealthy state, there had been an epidemic of hospital gangrene and to admit a badly burned patient would involve other operated cases in great danger'. The incident bore fruit for the Managers agreed to establish a small hospital for patients with burns. While Syme may not have seen in this the benefit of isolating the burnt patient from the risk of sepsis in the general ward, he at least recognised the danger of having such cases, which would inevitably become grossly infected, in contact with others in which there might be some hope of primary healing.[194]

Syme's reaction to Simpson's introduction of acupressure has already been described. Late in his life, however, his conservative notions began to be overthrown by the knowledge he derived from his continued and close association with his son-in-law. Syme as a practical surgeon eventually saw in Lister's antiseptic method an important advance in technique. Despite his extreme conservatism he accepted it and no doubt Lister had indoctrinated him gradually and tactfully.

Simpson saw Lister's discovery otherwise. He was deeply convinced that the theories on which he had based acupressure and with which he conducted his campaign on hospitalism were correct. He believed that by his work he was contributing to medicine and mankind advances which would ensure that his name would never be forgotten. To him acupressure was even more important than the discovery of the use of chloroform. We may look back and wonder why he did not rejoice at Lister's achievement and see in his teaching the things which had eluded him. Had Simpson accepted Lister's doctrines this would have enhanced his own efforts and put them in perspective. Simpson, however, failed (or some may say, refused) to grasp this opportunity. He was not alone in his disbelief for there were many of his stature and eminence who were equally unreceptive. It is inevitable that there should be an opinion that he was blinded by jealousy and that all the past animosities with Syme clouded his judgement. This may be partly true but in his last years, tempered perhaps by his religious beliefs, he showed an increasing desire to live at peace with his fellow men and to forgive past quarrels. By 1867 his intellectual powers may have declined to some extent from chronic ill-health and repeated acute illnesses, but this is belied by the energy which he displayed in his last years in furthering his own causes and in opposing Lister.

When Lister went to Glasgow he was appalled at the conditions in the wards of the Infirmary where excessive overcrowding was associated with a forbidding mortality from wound infection. He left Edinburgh with ideas very similar to those held by Syme but, unlike most surgeons who knew only the pathology of the late effects of inflammation, he had made an intensive study of the early phases of the process. From his investigations he had developed some scepticism towards established ideas. He questioned the theory that decomposition and consequent suppuration were set up by atmospheric influences. He knew that a patient with a severe limb fracture would escape the severe consequences of inflammation provided the skin was intact, but that with a compound fracture and a surface wound sepsis was almost inevitable and often fatal to limb if not life. For long he felt that if this difference could be explained the way would be open to the control of wound infection. When he learned of Pasteur's demonstration of the association of fermentation and putrefaction with micro-organisms, of his proof that such micro-organisms were carried in the air on particles of dust and of his ability to destroy micro-organisms by heat or chemicals, he had the answer to his problem. His practical application of Pasteur's findings to surgery is best repeated in his own words: [195]

But when it had been shown by the researches of Pasteur that the septic property of the atmosphere depended not upon oxygen, or any gaseous constituent but on minute organisms suspended in it, which owed their energy to their vitality, it occurred to me that decomposition in the injured part might be avoided without excluding the air, by applying as a dressing some material capable of destroying the life of the floating particles. . . .

The material I have employed is carbolic or phenic acid.

Lister heard of Pasteur's work in a chance conversation with the Professor of Chemistry in Glasgow early in 1865. Rather surprisingly he had not apparently seen reports which had already appeared in the British medical journals. There was, for example, a paper given by Spencer Wells at the annual meeting of the British Medical Association in Cambridge in August 1864. The subject was *Some causes of excessive mortality after surgical operations* and Wells not only referred in some detail to Pasteur's work but envisaged the possibility of controlling infections by a chemotherapeutic attack on bacteria. Wells missed his chance of immortality for he failed to see in Pasteur's observations the possibility, which Lister was to exploit, of preventing or controlling infection in surgery.

It was Lister's aim to prevent putrefaction or infection ever starting in a wound, this was his basic conception of antisepsis. He had to accept, however, that in many conditions such as compound fractures, with the wound contaminated by soil or other infected material, organisms were already implanted, He saw that he had to destroy these and prevent more entering the wound. Although he concentrated largely in eliminating the risks of inoculation from bacteria carried in the air, he recognised also the necessity of destroying organisms on instruments, on the surgeons' hands, on the patients' skin and on dressings. Pasteur had used heat to destroy bacteria but this was impracticable for living tissues. Lister chose, from many possible agents, carbolic acid as a chemical antiseptic. To test his hypothesis he applied the new technique in the treatment of compound fractures. He did not really need any controls for this clinical experiment because the consistently disastrous results of treatment for such conditions were all too well known in every hospital. He cleaned the wound, mopped out all the crevices with a piece of lint soaked in undiluted carbolic acid and then applied a dressing soaked in the acid. The dressing was sealed with plaster and covered by a thin metal plate. The plate was removed from time to time and the outer part of the dressing resoaked with carbolic. After a few days the dressing was removed to reveal a tenacious crust or scab on the wound and there was seldom any suppuration. Lister was cautious and he delayed publication of his results until 1867 when he was able to record that of 11 major compound fractures so treated 9 had survived with life and limb. One patient died from a haemorrhage unassociated with sepsis and one required a delayed amputation for gangrene. The series was small but the results were remarkable and the efficacy of the antiseptic treatment was established in his mind. Lister spent the rest of his active surgical life improving his techniques and trying out different antiseptics but his principles remained unchanged. His pre-occupation with air-borne infection led to the development of the spray, a cumbersome and ineffective device which in time he discarded. More important was his introduction in 1868 of the sterile cat-gut ligature, for this eliminated immediately the need for the long ligature, the risk of infection from traditional materials less readily sterilised than cat-gut, Simpson's finicky acupressure needles and Wells' clumsy ovariotomy clamp.

Lister's case was nearly unassailable but there was one weakness. He had taken a gamble in accepting the germ theory of disease and at this stage he offered no proof, by the microscope or otherwise, that organisms in the air were identical with those found in a suppurating wound. This final confirmation was to come later with more exact techniques, such as the specific staining of organisms and the use of cultures. Although the germ theory of disease had been gaining ground since the Italian Bassi had, as early as 1825, demonstrated that a silk-worm disease was caused by a microscopic fungus, there was still in 1867 a deeply ingrained belief in the theory of spontaneous generation of micro-organisms and even of higher forms of life. The theory had the support of Cuvier and other influential scientists. After Pasteur published his work he was challenged by Pouchet who denied the validity of his experiments. It was not until 1865 that the French Academy reported in favour of Pasteur. Lister had in fact accepted a concept which was unproven. There were, not surprisingly, many who considered that Lister's reasoning was based, therefore, on an inaccurate premise. In Edinburgh Dr Hughes Bennet gave, in January 1868, a lecture on the 'atmospheric germ theory', in which he acknowledged the early dictum of Harvey *omne vivium ex ovo* for the higher forms of life, but denied its application to the lower forms of life such as fungi and other micro-organisms. He supported Pouchet's defence of spontaneous generation and his refutation of Pasteur's work. Bennet developed his arguments from a long series of personal experiments on parasitic organisms. From the illustrations in his text it is clear that he had been misled because of his primitive microscopic technique. This was nevertheless a reasoned criticism of the foundations on which Lister had based his principles. It was otherwise with the majority of Lister's antagonists for they did not attack the principles but devoted their energies to criticism of his choice of carbolic acid, ignoring the fact that he had stressed that he might well have chosen some other 'anti-septic' substance. To many Lister's method was quite simply equated with the local dressing of wounds by carbolic acid and they failed to see that he used the term antisepsis in an original manner. Carbolic acid in one form or another was not new in therapeutics. In 1859 Calvert had shown its value in the preservation of anatomical material and recommended its use to surgeons as a wound dressing. In France, Lemaire had published a whole book about its therapeutic properties in 1863. Lister was accused by many of a false and even dishonest claim of priority in the use of carbolic. It is rather distressing to find that Simpson appears so prominently amongst those who attacked Lister on such grounds. The conflict between him and Lister can be followed best by recording the proceedings of the annual meetings of the British Medical Association in 1867 and 1869, at Dublin and Leeds respectively.[196]

At Dublin the annual address on surgery was given by Robert Smith. In most of these addresses the progress of surgery was reviewed and the more imaginative speakers were bold enough to forecast future developments. Too often,

however, the surgeon selected took the opportunity of recalling his personal contributions or of riding some private
hobby-horse. Smith was no exception to this for he devoted
most of his paper to a rather dull discussion of his views on
certain bone injuries. He did not even mention Lister who
had just published his epoch-making papers. There was one
reference to Simpson's acupressure and this was only to bring
forward some rather obscure evidence that, far from being
original, the method had been described in the sixteenth
century by John de Vigo.[197]

Pirrie of Aberdeen read a paper on acupressure. He was one
of the few remaining enthusiastic supporters of the technique
and he gave a favourable account. In the discussion which
followed Simpson first of all took the chance of contradicting
Smith's statement that acupressure had been invented two
centuries previously. (He sent a long paper the very next week
to the *British Medical Journal* enlarging on this subject and
castigating Smith for his careless translation of de Vigo's
Latin.) He was delighted at Pirrie's support and emphasised
further the favourable influence of acupressure on wound
healing. He then made reference to the antiseptic method
and on this occasion at least he showed he had given some
thought to the principles involved for he said: 'No one has
yet, I believe, seen these mythical fungi with the eye or with
the microscope'. This solitary sentence has been quoted as
proving that Simpson did not believe in the existence of
micro-organisms but in the context he implied that, for
wound infection at least, the germ theory of disease was still
unproven. There is no record that Lister was present at this
discussion but he was in Dublin and at the last minute a paper
by him *On the Antiseptic Principle in the Practice of Surgery*,
was added to the programme of the surgical section. He gave a
concise account of his methods and summarised the results
he had published in the *Lancet* earlier in the year. There
was one important addition for he said: 'When the antiseptic
treatment is efficiently conducted, ligatures may be safely
cut short and left to be disposed of by absorption or otherwise.'
Although in due course the paper was published in full in
the journal, it is interesting to note that in the immediate
reports of the meeting there was no mention even that it had

been on the programme. There was a discussion after the paper but this is learned about only from remarks which Simpson makes in a subsequent article on carbolic acid, to which reference is made below. All we know is that Professor Hingston of Montreal criticised Lister adversely and that Simpson, 'amongst other remarks', drew attention to the use of carbolic acid in surgery in France and Germany before 1865 and denied that Lister had produced anything that was new. It cannot be said that the delegates who heard Lister's paper went home with a feeling that history had been made and that surgery was on the brink of a revolution.[198]

When Simpson returned to Edinburgh, having polished off Smith for his rather pointless reference to acupressure, he got down to the business of attacking Lister. Early in September a letter appeared in the *Edinburgh Daily Review* signed 'Chirurgicus'. There is every reason to believe that Simpson was the writer. Once more Lister was accused of having claimed unjustly an originality in the use of carbolic acid and the priority was given to Lemaire. The *Lancet* quoted this letter and Lister, usually so reluctant to enter a quarrel, felt constrained to write to the editor and complain that he should have taken note of an anonymous letter in the lay press. He admitted he had not seen Lemaire's book but he did not think it important because he knew that in Paris no one had instituted a system of antiseptic treatment such as his. He finally referred to his paper at the Dublin meeting and the 'feeble attempt to decry it as useless'. He had probably no doubt about Simpson being the author of the attack. Simpson soon came out in the open with a long article *Carbolic Acid and its Compounds in Surgery*. In this he gave a list of those who had used carbolic acid previously and suggested that Lemaire had anticipated Lister, not only in his choice of antiseptic but in the principles of its employment. The real message comes at the end of the article:[199]

> One great and most laudable object which Professor Lister evidently has in view in using carbolic acid as a local dressing is to close these wounds entirely by the first intention and without any suppuration. . . . But these paramount objects have been attained in the hospital of Aberdeen by the use of acupressure.

Simpson must now have recognised that Lister's work was beginning to distract attention from acupressure. It was not a very convincing paper but Lister could scarcely ignore it. He replied to the accusations with quiet dignity.[200]

> The elaborate communication of Sir James Simpson in today's *Lancet* may seem to require some reply. But as I have already endeavoured to place the matter in its true light without doing injustice to anyone, I must forbear from any comment, on his allegations. . . . I have arranged to publish, with your permission, a series of papers explanatory of the subject in question, and your readers will then be able to judge for themselves how far the present attack admits of justification.

The Leeds meeting was two years later. Simpson meanwhile produced his elaborate statistics on hospitalism. Lister had greatly strengthened his case by publishing further convincing results using modifications of his original technique. He had, in addition, now introduced sterile cat-gut which, as has been noted, was of exceptional importance in surgery.

Simpson knew that the annual address on surgery was to be given by Thomas Nunneley (1809-1870), a Leeds surgeon of some authority and eminence. He knew also that Nunneley was antagonistic to Lister's ideas. Perhaps he felt this was his last chance to impress on the medical world his passionate views on hospitalism and his absolute faith in acupressure. He wrote to Nunneley on the 18th July, 1869, two weeks before the meeting: [201]

> How is your address developing itself? I wish anxiously to get up to Leeds to hear it and three papers on the list about the construction of Hospitals and Hospitalism. But I fear I shall not be able to escape. The Countess of Kintail has come here to have a child in the last ten days of July and to have chloroform which her London doctors some years have refused to give—as she had a loud cardiac bruit. If she is better in time I will run off; if not I am fixed here.
>
> You told me you intended *inter alia* to discuss the mortality of amputations in Hospitals. I have 11 or 12,000 limb amputations from Provincial Hospitals reported to me, with a total mortality of about 1 in 4. . . .
>
> I have a case near me here which I wish I could shew you. The operation—excision of the cancerous mamma, was performed 10 days ago. I had to use three needles which were

soon removed. . . . The wound—a long one has united entirely without one single drop of pus. No dressings used. *No* carbolic acid. Was there ever a higher delusion than seeing men—rational men anointing their knives and saws with it. . . .

The statistics of amputations and of compound fractures are worse, I believe, in the Glasgow and Edinburgh Hospitals since it was used there—than before it. . . . In an operation 40 or 50 years ago at which your townsman Mr Hey was present the femoral artery was tied with cat-gut, the ends cut off and the wound healed entirely by the first intention. But the cat-gut was not carbolised. When the *same* result follows in 1869 and the cat-gut *is* carbolised the result is illogically attributed to the carbolic acid instead of the ligature.

Simpson was able to travel to Leeds in time for the meeting but Lister was not present. In the opening address the President, Charles Chadwick, described the new hospital which had just been built in Leeds. It incorporated in its design many of the things to which Simpson had taken exception. Chadwick thought Simpson was wrong in most of his ideas and he rubbed salt into the wound when he said that in any case Lister's work would diminish hospital infection. The address on surgery by Nunneley was tedious in the extreme and after a long and disjointed review of operative surgery the more controversial subjects were introduced. There was a brief reference to acupressure which was dismissed as of limited value and this must have been a disappointment to Simpson. Finally Nunneley made a prolonged and ill-devised attack on Lister: [202]

> The sound physiological and pathological doctrines of the last generation of British surgeons are unheeded, and in danger of being temporarily forgotten for what seem to me unsupported fancies, which have little other existence than what is found in the imagination of those who believe in them. . . . If the antiseptic theory be true no wound ought ever to have healed until carbolic acid or some like substance, had been discovered and applied.

He continued with a jumble of unrelated facts and fancies about wound healing. He quoted Pouchet and Hughes Bennet in an attempt to render the germ theory of disease ridiculous. He had not understood Lister's writings and he had not even seen his methods used. He affirmed that while he in the last three years had never used carbolic acid some of his fellow surgeons in Leeds had tried it and then given it up. This statement was challenged and Nunneley was heavily criticised for his inaccuracy. If Simpson had hoped that Nunneley would deliver a death-blow to Listerism he was soon mistaken.

Lister wrote another of his short but crushing letters when the speech was reported in the journals: [203]

> Mr Nunneley's recent attack seems to me little calculated to impede the progress of the antiseptic treatment: nor do I feel called upon to point out in how many reports he has misapprehended my published views. That he should dogmatically oppose a treatment which he so little understands and which by his own admission, he has never tried, is a matter of small moment. But I was grieved to find him stating that his colleagues who had once adopted the system, were now abandoning it as untrustworthy. It was therefore with much pleasure that I received a different account of the matter in a letter which, with his permission, I now request you to publish.

Nunneley's confusion and prejudice were typical of many of Lister's opponents and although the association journal reported his speech as one of 'outspoken and honest criticism, founded on observation and experience' there were many who thought differently. Lister was right in believing that in the end such opinions would be ignored. Although Simpson must have felt that Nunneley had failed in his attempt to discredit Lister, he may have derived some comfort in the support he received when there was a full discussion on hospital construction. A Captain Galton read a paper on this subject and in it he supported many of Simpson's views. In the discussion which followed, Dr Evory Kennedy, who was now a distinguished obstetrician in Dublin and had been Simpson's main rival for the Edinburgh Chair, went far towards agreement. Simpson spoke and took the opportunity of expressing his iconoclastic views as strongly as ever. He reported that despite Lister's claims of the benefits of antisepsis the Glasgow and Edinburgh hospitals were having just as high a mortality in amputations as in the past. Macleod of Glasgow defended his colleagues and felt that Simpson's statistics were a misrepresentation of the position. However, in some support of Simpson, he quoted his experience in the Crimean War when he had worked in a hutted hospital which he had found ideal. Holmes Coote of London frankly condemned both the concept of hospitalism and Listerism, believing implicitly that hospital infection was due to the inhalation of 'animal poisons'. Dr Acland and some others were very concerned that Simpson's insistence on the dangers of large hospitals would alarm an undiscerning public, so that not only would they be afraid to come into hospital as patients but also they would stop subscribing to the support of these voluntary organisations. There was a great deal of confusion in the minds of most of those who participated in the debate but in general there was an acceptance of many of Simpson's views.

From 1849, when Simpson first gave his views on the dangers of large hospitals, on the desirability of treating patients in small isolated units built in the country and on the merits of using methods of construction so that replacement was economical and rapid, he wrote many papers on the subject. There was plenty of general evidence to support his views. From time to time the surgical wards of large hospitals were overwhelmed with epidemics of erysipelas, hospital gangrene or pyaemia so that there was no alternative but to close them, fumigate them and wash down the walls with chloride of lime in the hope that some mysterious miasma would be eradicated. Some thought that these outbreaks would be solved by improving ventilation and increasing the circulation of a purer air; others thought there was too much ventilation. Simpson was greatly impressed by military experience in various campaigns when it had been shown that results were better, as far as sepsis was concerned, in tented hospitals or in temporary hutments. He knew about the disasters of overcrowding and lack of hygiene which occurred in the huge barrack hospitals of Scutari during the Crimean War. In 1855, in an attempt to provide safer hospital accommodation for the sick and wounded, the War Office asked the engineer Isambard Brunel to design a new kind of hospital to be erected in a healthy site at Renkioi on the shores of the Dardanelles. It consisted of a series of pre-fabricated wooden huts with carefully planned ventilation systems, washing and toilet facilities and bed space (which compare well with many modern hospitals). With astonishing speed Brunel defied governmental red tape and produced the plans within 10 days. In six months the units were shipped out to the East and the hospital was receiving its first patients. It never worked to full capacity but those like Spencer Wells who served in it while attached to the army as civilian surgeons were convinced of its merits. Although there is no proof that Simpson had a hand in this design it certainly embodied some of his ideas. He received a copy of the final report prepared by Dr Parkes, who superintended its construction and its operation.[204]

Simpson felt that he had to prove his arguments by statistics and for more than 10 years he laboured at this task. He chose to survey the results of major amputations done in different environments. With immense labour he collected mortality rates from the major hospitals in the British Isles and, for comparison, he obtained the results of amputations done either in patients' homes or in small country cottage hospitals. By 1869 his final figures showed that of 2,089 amputations done in hospital practice 855 died, while of 2,098 done in country practice only 26 died. The bare statement of these figures does not even hint at the trouble he took to support his case, in his careful analysis of the details of each case and in the production of endless comparative tables for specific operations or for individual hospitals. To Simpson the evidence was incontrovertible but to others it remained unconvincing. The most valid criticism was that although it was relatively easy to acquire large series of reasonably accurate figures from individual hospitals, it was quite a different matter to take a large number of single cases, or at most small groups of cases, from individual country practitioners who did not always keep accurate records, who depended on their memory alone and who, being human, would tend to forget their failures. Despite this undoubted weakness the figures were startling and Simpson may be excused for becoming impatient and irate at those who refused to be stirred by his conclusions. To many surgeons Simpson's attacks on the hospital system were taken as a reflection on their work and as a personal affront. When Simpson addressed the Association for the Promotion of Social Science in 1867 and expounded his views to the laity, there was a genuine fear that the frail

economic system of voluntary support for the great hospitals
would collapse.[205]

Few topics in these years gave rise to so much discussion and
argument as did hospitalism. Amongst the many antagonists
was Thomas Holmes, surgeon to St George's Hospital. He
presented a paper with fair criticism of Simpson's amputation
statistics and he concluded by discussing the results following
operations in the great metropolitan hospitals: [206]

> Much of the mortality I believe to be inevitable: still it is a
> most important question whether all of it is so. I recognise most
> fully the service which Sir J. Y. Simpson is doing in bringing
> this question publicly forward: and although I cannot avoid
> differing from his conclusions, I do full justice to the noble
> and charitable motives which have prompted the investiga-
> tion.

Holmes, like so many others, accepted that there was
something inevitable about hospital mortality and it was this
defeatist attitude which Simpson wanted to overcome. Not all
the critics were as generous as Holmes was in his tribute to
Simpson's honesty and deep sense of mission. Syme, not unexpectedly, entered the lists after Holmes' paper appeared: [207]

> For some time past the London medical journals and Edin-
> burgh newspapers have been the vehicles of a persevering
> attempt to shake public confidence in large hospitals, on the
> grounds that operations in them are less successful than those
> performed on patients in their own residences however poor
> and uncomfortable. But all the copious and unscrupulous
> statements adduced in support of this might very well have
> been spared; since the observations of military surgeons dur-
> ing the Peninsular campaigns completely established the fact
> that operations, and especially amputations, have a much less
> chance of recovery in crowded divisional hospitals than when
> performed on the field. . . .

He went on to argue the necessity of providing large hospitals so that patients could have the benefit of concentrated
medical care and of comforts which would not be available
in their homes. He did not see how instruction could be given
to students without the concentration of large numbers of
cases. In his opinion the alleged dangers could be obviated not
by changes in ventilation or by drastic schemes of reconstruc-

tion, but by ensuring that beds should be more than three feet apart. He went back to his earlier years when in 1833 he had solved the problems of infection in the surgical wards of the converted High School by insisting on a reduction of the number of beds. Avoidance of overcrowding and the application of the antiseptic system were, in his opinion, the simple solutions.

When Syme wrote this letter there was a considerable argument raging about the site and style of a new Edinburgh Royal Infirmary. Syme was dissatisfied with the existing surgical accommodation which had not been in use for very long. He advocated that a comprehensive new hospital should be built on a site to be vacated by George Watson's Hospital School. He had been accused of having opposed the transfer of the old Infirmary to this new site but gave sound reasons for his change of opinion. One objection was that the new hospital would be some distance from the medical school and that the students would take 15 to 20 minutes to get there. Syme had measured the distance and found he could walk it in three minutes. In one of his rare flashes of humour he said that the students could do the same provided they did not stop on the way for a glass of beer and a cigar! Simpson, not unexpectedly, recommended that they should build a series of small readily replaceable buildings instead of a huge monumental single block. There was no comment on this suggestion. By 1876 the present Infirmary was completed incorporating the advantages and the disadvantages of hospital construction as recommended by Miss Florence Nightingale.

While Simpson was fighting his rather hopeless rearguard action in support of acupressure and, with rather more encouragement, pushing forward his views on hospitalism, Syme was quietly becoming aware of the significance of Lister's work. Syme's influence was powerful, not only in Edinburgh but throughout the whole country, and that he did eventually come forward in support of the antiseptic method was of great importance to Lister's cause. In July 1867 he sent to the *Lancet* a brief paper: *On the treatment of incised wounds with a view to union by the first intention.* He described Lister's practice as 'certainly the most important improvement in surgical practice of recent times'. He reported three cases in which he had used carbolic acid in the approved manner but said more about the value of torsion to control bleeding vessels than about the new dressing technique. Perhaps he was still a little wary of accepting all that he had been told by his son-in-law. His caution was relaxed, however, soon after these early trials and in January 1868 he published a short paper *Illustrations of the antiseptic principle of treatment in surgery*. He described seven cases in which he had used the method with success and showed a full appreciation of the principles involved. He explained the bad results reported from London by a failure of the practitioners concerned to see that there was something more than just a carbolic acid dressing: [208]

> The Truth is, that the antiseptic system, in order to be employed with advantage, must be carefully studied and fully understood, theoretically as well as practically. . . .
>
> Some attempts have been made anonymously and otherwise, to filch away from Mr Lister the credit justly due to him for devising and establishing the antiseptic system, by representing the use of carbolic acid previously for other purposes as an anticipation of his treatment. But, although the agent was not new the principles of its employment, the modes of its application, and the results of its effects, being so entirely original, I venture to hope that the members of my profession will no longer tacitly sanction such disingenuous and ungenerous conduct.

It cannot be said that Syme supported Lister with excessive enthusiasm but age and ill-health had taken their toll and he had lost his zest for argument. Some may suggest that he climbed on the band-waggon at the last possible minute. It may be wondered if, had it not been for his close relationship to Lister or his antagonism to Simpson, he might well have ranged himself with Nunneley and all the other disbelievers. Syme, however, had a keen analytical mind and he should be credited with having developed, if slowly, a full appreciation of the importance of the antiseptic doctrine. In a letter of February 1869 he showed some understanding of the difficulties encountered by Lister in putting over his case and advised him: 'Instead of "antiseptic" I think you should call the system of treatment "protective" to avoid confusion. . . .'

Further, his sense of justice was so strongly ingrained that, had he not believed in Lister's work, family considerations would not have swayed him.[209]

It is a somewhat tragic reflection that Simpson, who strived so hard to solve the problem of hospital infection, should have derived so little credit. His work was overshadowed by Lister's ultimate success in establishing his principles. If Simpson failed it was a magnificent failure and in retrospect he deserves much more recognition than has hitherto been granted to him. He impressed on his profession the urgent need for action in an attempt to eliminate, or at least diminish, the cruel complications of sepsis. He shook the surgeons out of their complacency.

CHAPTER 11

Last Years

IN their last years the two professors continued in practice with unremitting energy and the flow of lectures and case reports to the journals was unabated.

Syme broke new ground with more advanced techniques in the treatment of aneurysms and tumours. In 1861 he tied the iliac artery for a huge gluteal aneurysm, 'a bold operation not seen for 60 years'. There was still some of the drama of the pre-anaesthetic era and he had lost none of his expertise. The *Lancet* described the alarming gushes of blood which shattered the audience but in no way discomposed Mr Syme. Faced with torrential bleeding he remained cool and controlled the situation by laying open the huge distended blood vessel. The audience greeted his success with loud applause (such uninhibited demonstrations always displeased him). There was another exciting occasion when he dealt with the equally difficult problem of an iliac aneurysm. For this operation Lister came from Glasgow to assist and brought his new and fearsome tourniquet by which pressure was exerted through the abdominal wall to control the aorta. In 1865, after many previous failures, Syme succeeded in removing the whole of the tongue for cancer, an operation fraught with great risk. Such achievements were recognised even in London as evidence of his continued masterly skill.

In this decade, although Simpson was so heavily involved in his work on acupressure and hospitalism, he made further advances in obstetrics and gynaecology. His lectures covered the whole of these subjects and editors vied with each other for the privilege of printing them. His assistants did much of the writing and he himself never had the time to produce a full text-book.

Few contemporary problems were ignored and both Syme and Simpson had little hesitation in expressing their views on subjects outside their immediate interests. Simpson was criticised for his interference in purely surgical matters when he introduced acupressure. Syme did not escape censure either, as when he made a sweeping condemnation of the operation of iridectomy for glaucoma and pronounced this disease incurable. The ophthalmic surgeon Bowman and his colleagues attacked Syme vigorously for his statements, affirming that he was terrified of anything new and questioning his ability to give an opinion on something of which he had no experience.

When the Siamese twins visited Great Britain in 1869 they went to Edinburgh to consult both professors. The twins were now decrepit and aged and each had a horror of the other dying. Syme gave his opinion briefly and tersely, that no attempt should be made at separation. This was the advice already firmly given by Nélaton in Paris and Fergusson in London. Simpson, his curiosity as lively as ever, went more deeply into the question for he had always been interested in deformities and double monsters. He persuaded Chang and Eng to be demonstrated to his class when he gave a lecture on the subject of conjoined twins. He said that the brothers did not wish to be separated but that some of their relatives were pressing for this to be done. There were awkward domestic complications because one had become estranged from his wife! Simpson investigated the connection between the two at the upper abdominal level and tried to find out the contents of the band by shining a powerful electric light through it. He did not think any important organs such as the liver were joined but advised against operation on the grounds that it would be justified only for 'seemliness and convenience' and not as a matter of life and death. He did an ingenious experiment to estimate the extent of the cross-circulation of blood. Eng obliged by swallowing 10 grains of potassium iodide and an hour later Chang obliged by passing a specimen of urine which was shown to contain iodide. Simpson published his lecture in full with one of his detailed historical reviews in which he illustrated the classic cases of conjoined twins over the centuries. Perhaps he would dearly have loved to operate on the twins but he was wise not to do so because with all the publicity attendant on their progress through Europe a fatality would have been widely criticised.[210]

The attitude of the two men towards animal experiment in medical research is of some interest. Syme early in his career had done such experiments when he studied the growth of bone but thereafter he showed little enthusiasm. He most likely saw dangers in the uncontrolled and increasing popularity of the technique and, in addition, there were murmurs from the anti-vivisectionists. He thought it quite unnecessary for students to repeat in their training the basic experiments from which lessons had already been clearly drawn. In 1868 he tried to have accepted 'that the use of living animals shall as far as possible be avoided in teaching and in scientific research'. Simpson, in contrast, was a confirmed believer in animal experiment. As early as 1837 he had co-operated with Henry Imlach in a study of softening, erosion and perforation of the stomach. They had fed animals with various chemicals and had even studied the effect on the stomach of division of the vagus nerve in the cat and the rabbit. In his work on anaesthesia and acupressure all sorts of animals from eels to horses were used. Some of these experiments may have been haphazard but Simpson did understand the necessity of having controls. It is never quite clear where he did all this work for there is no mention of a laboratory. Some may have been done in the stables behind his house in Queen Street and he had friends in the country who may have looked after all the rabbits, cats, dogs, pigs and even larger animals which he used. Simpson seems to have escaped the attentions of the anti-vivisectionists. Like many scientists who accept the necessity of experimenting on living creatures he was intensely fond of animals, as is testified by the succession of much loved dogs which were part of the Simpson household.[211]

The affairs of the University continued in an uneasy atmosphere, particularly as far as professorial appointments were concerned. In 1864 Professor Miller died and Lister made his first attempt to return to Edinburgh. He was defeated by Spence by one vote and Syme no doubt did his best to get his son-in-law appointed. Simpson was accused of intrigue when

Laycock succeeded Alison in the Chair of Medicine. Over all these appointments attempts were made to revive the Test Act and there was heated discussion over the religious beliefs of prospective candidates.[212]

In 1863 Elizabeth Garret Anderson came to Edinburgh in the hope of being admitted to medical classes in the University. Simpson gave her some help by arranging that she should receive instruction in midwifery under his colleague Keiller. Simpson was sympathetic towards these brave pioneers and his influence may have had something to do with Edinburgh's acceptance of women students, after a period of considerable dissension, earlier than other medical schools. The majority of the professors maintained a united front against this terrible intrusion for several years. Syme's views are not recorded but it seems likely that he disapproved of the idea of women becoming doctors.[213]

In February 1868 Sir David Brewster, Principal of the University, died. Prior to 1858 the position had been held by a succession of men who were usually Professors of Divinity and members of the established Church of Scotland and some exerted considerable control and beneficial influence. By the University Act of 1858 the powers of the Principal were more clearly defined and he acted as Chairman of both Senate and Council. The salary was meagre at £700 a year but usually a house was provided. In 1858 Dr John Lee had been succeeded by Brewster who had made a great reputation as a scientist by his work in optics. He had invented the kaleidoscope and devised a new and improved method for the illumination for lighthouses. He had some literary reputation from his biography of Isaac Newton. Accepted internationally as the doyen of the scientific world, he had been for 21 years Principal of St Andrew's University. He was already 78 when he came to Edinburgh but served there for 8 years with tact and ability: 'a determined lover of peace, a wise ruler, respected by all his subjects, and a delightful companion'. With all these virtues and his international fame it was not easy to find a worthy successor.[214]

Before Brewster died he had expressed the hope that he would be succeeded by Professor Christison. Although already aged 71 Christison was in many ways an ideal candidate, experienced in University affairs, popular with students and staff and remarkably active mentally and physically. After some thought he declined to be nominated. The names of Syme, Simpson and Playfair, Professor of Chemistry, were put forward from Edinburgh. There were at least two outside candidates, Sir Alexander Grant of Bombay and Allen Thomson, Professor of Anatomy in Glasgow. The candidature of Syme was never seriously considered. By the end of March, with the withdrawal of Christison, it was clear that the choice lay between Simpson and Grant. Thus was initiated an election in which the supporters of both men were to exhibit an unparalleled degree of dissension, bitterness and deceit. The official University Minutes concerning the election are, perhaps not surprisingly, silent concerning this affair. There is, however, a wealth of information in contemporary newspapers and medical journals and in Simpson's papers.

Sir Alexander Grant (1826-1884) had in 1863 been appointed Vice-Chancellor of the University of Bombay and was in India when he was nominated for the Principalship. He was the seventh holder of a Baronetcy of Nova Scotia, created in 1688. Born in New York he had been educated at Harrow and Oxford. His academic reputation rested on his *Ethics of Aristotle*, published when he was in Oxford in 1857. There were mixed opinions about the merit of this work but he had been very successful as an administrator and educationalist in India. Initially he was interested in the Chair of Moral Philosophy in Edinburgh and when the Principalship became vacant he aspired to both appointments.[215]

There was much skirmishing by interested parties and enquiries were initiated about Grant's character, his academic background and, most of all, his religious beliefs. Opinion was sought from Oxford and the replies varied: 'Grant is liberal in his religious views and broadchurch'; 'His Aristotle indifferent, his religious opinions free and unsettled'; 'Broadchurchman—does not hold the Inspiration of Scripture, the necessity of Christ's death as an atonement for sin . . . and other kindred errors'. Many had doubts about the propriety of appointing one of the persuasion of the Church of England, however 'broad' he might be. To some a Harrow and Oxford education seemed inappropriate for the Principal of Edinburgh University. Although Grant came of a Scottish family his only connection with Edinburgh was in his marriage to the grand-daughter of Professor Wilson (the greatly esteemed Christopher North). To a majority Grant's qualifications did not seem outstanding. His support was to come as much from those who were against Simpson as from those who really believed he was an ideal choice.

It is said that Simpson was reluctant to stand for the Principalship. Certainly in early April he wrote to his former assistant Dr Watt Black: [216]

> ... the public, not myself, have set me forward as a candidate for the Principalship; but I have not yet applied, Professor Christison, Syme, Playfair etc. all started. But I believe it lies at present between me and Sir A. Grant of Bombay, who will not take it unless he gets the vacant Moral Philosophy Chair also. The time of the election is not fixed, and I will not be greatly disappointed if it does not fall on me.

Whatever his early feelings may have been it is clear from Simpson's letters and other documents that once the contest developed he was not only hopeful of success but he very definitely wanted the appointment. He had a great love for the University and to him the Principalship was a prize which would have sealed the success of his career. In many ways he was well equipped. He had always taken a great interest in the welfare of his students and in the affairs of all the faculties. He had been a remarkably successful ambassador for the University at home and abroad and he had international fame. No one could deny the importance of his contributions to medical science and his antiquarian research enhanced his academic status. He could count on overwhelming support from the medical profession and he had powerful friends in other walks of life. The medical journals were almost unanimously on his side and some regarded his election as a foregone conclusion. He must have been aware that there would be strong opposition from those on the Senate who had always been against him but it seems unlikely that he expected quite such crushing opposition as that which came from this quarter. At no time was there any statement about the necessity of his relinquishing the Chair of Obstetrics should he have been appointed Principal, but it may be surmised that he was prepared to give this up or retain it in some modified form provided he was allowed to continue in private practice.

The election was in the hands of the Curators of the University. This body consisted of seven members of whom three were elected by the University and four by the City Council. At one moment the Curators were said to be in favour of Simpson, at the next in favour of Grant. On June 10th there was a premature announcement that Simpson had already been chosen. The final decision was to be taken towards the end of June but at the last minute the meeting was postponed. Seldom had rumours been more conflicting but in these months there happened a series of incidents which determined the final result.

By the end of April there was an increasing support for Grant but not everyone seemed clear as to whether he sought the Chair of Moral Philosophy, the Principalship or both these appointments. Grant's promoters were well aware of the strength of Simpson's candidature and of the doubts and aspersions which had been cast on Grant's academic achievements and on his religious beliefs.

Scarcely had the campaign got going than the rival faction issued a printed document in which Simpson was accused of spreading rumours about Grant's indifference to religion. It was alleged that Mr Campbell Duns had discussed with Simpson the merits of Grant's qualifications and that Simpson had suggested that information should be sought directly from Bombay. A telegram was despatched by Duns to Mr Brown in Bombay, the son of the Rev. Dr Brown of Edinburgh. It was terse and to the point: 'Is Sir A. Grant a Broad Churchman and indifferent lecturer? Candidate for Moral Philosophy Chair'. Back came the reply: 'An indifferent Churchman. Broad religious views. A popular lecturer. Caution in the use of this'. It was alleged that Simpson received this telegram directly and that he used it to further his own cause.

The reply had, in fact, come to Duns and he had shown it to Simpson. It is likely at this stage that Simpson, deeply involved as usual in the choice of a new professor, was genuinely concerned about Grant's suitability to teach moral philosophy. Those unfavourably disposed towards Simpson

227

who heard of the exchange of telegrams believed however that
he had employed underhand methods for his own advantage.
It is significant that by the end of April some of his friends
wrote to him withdrawing their support. The effect of this
incident was trivial compared with all that was to follow.

On or about May 7th Syme, undoubtedly a leader of the
opposition to Simpson, sent a letter to Gibson Craig one of the
Curators representing the University. The document was
given to the Clerk to read out at the next meeting of the
Curators and then it was destroyed. It is clear that something
was divulged which proved gravely detrimental to Simpson.
Repeated attempts were made by Simpson and his supporters
to find out the contents of the letter but with no success.
Syme was approached but refused to divulge what he had
written although at one stage he denied that he had defamed
Simpson's character. There must have been more in the letter
than was to be repeated in the public attack on Simpson from
his fellow professors and from anonymous enemies who wrote
to the newspapers. There is a draft in Simpson's hand of a
letter to Adam Black dated June 18th: [217]

> Lord Provost stated that a letter from one of the Professors
> stated that I was not on speaking terms with many of my
> colleagues. Was this true? . . . Betimes I heard that the letter
> was written by Syme to Sir William Craig. I called on him
> and told above—I heard of *other* contents of letter. Wrote to
> Craig asking for a copy. Craig had burned letter and would
> not remember contents (conveniently).

Before this incident Adam Black, a City Council repre-
sentative, was a supporter of Simpson but at the final election
Black voted against Simpson. At this stage Sir William Gibson
Craig was in favour of Grant.

Was Syme malicious enough to use his knowledge of the
case of Mrs Q., to which reference has been made, and to
hint to the Curators that Simpson had fathered an illegitimate
child? It was certainly about this time that Mrs Q. may have
communicated her dark suspicions to Syme and others. Whatever Syme wrote in the letter caused considerable embarrass-
ment to the Curators and they did everything they could to
hush up the matter.

On June 12th the Reverend Blackie sent a letter to Baillie

Fyfe, another of the Curators elected by the City. He wrote in support of Grant: [218]

I believe he would raise the University in renown and specially adequately represent it among scholars and scholarly men in particular, which Sir James Simpson would never do: his powers of administration would be put forth to the greatest advantage, in these times when changes are undoubtedly required: while in a moral and religious point of view, his influence, aided by that of so decided and admirable a Christian woman as Lady Grant, would quietly but powerfully tend for good. . . . On the other hand though Sir James Simpson speaks more about religion, his religious character is destitute of solidarity and his moral texture is strangely and not to say loosely compacted. I fear the students would not respect him and the Professors will not work along with him. In his own sphere he is worthy of all honour, but I feel that his appointment as Principal would be a very serious mistake.

The letter was perfectly reasonable as an expression of opinion and no doubt many similar letters for or against both candidates were sent to the Curators. Whether or not the assessment of Simpson's moral and religious character amounted to slander is perhaps questionable. What mattered was the curious fate of the letter. Blackie gave it to his son Walter to be delivered by hand to Fyfe. Walter did not go direct to Fyfe's house but called on Professor Fraser on the way. He left the letter at Fraser's house for an hour and by a strange coincidence Professor Christison arrived at this very moment! Both Christison and Fraser read the letter and had it copied. It was then sent to other Curators and one of them, Milne Hume, thought it an excellent plan to show it to Simpson's friends. Later Professor Christison tried to persuade Simpson to withdraw from the election in view of the opinions expressed by Blackie. Although the letter did not influence Baillie Fyfe it must have spread doubts in the minds of those who were as yet undecided.

On June 17th a memorial was sent to the Curators from 12 members of the Senate: [219]

We the undersigned Members of the Senatus Academicus, having heard with regret that it is the intention of the Curators to appoint our colleague Sir James Simpson to the office of Principal of the University, and having reason to believe that the Curators are proceeding under the impression that his appointment would be acceptable to the Senatus generally, deem it our duty to express the conviction that it would not be for the advantage of the University.

It was not surprising to find Syme, Fraser and Christison amongst the signatories. There was also Piazzi Smyth who had not recovered from Simpson's attack on his theory about the pyramids! Simpson must have been saddened to find his old friend Douglas Maclagan against him. This was by no means a majority of the professors but Syme and Christison, in particular, were men of great influence.

As the election approached anonymous letters began to appear in the Edinburgh newspapers. On July 1st the *Courant* published a letter signed 'Civis' in which Simpson was attacked. His quarrel with Professor Piazzi Smyth was deplored, he had no business acumen, he was hostile to his students and he was unlikely to entertain in the style expected of a Principal. On July 3rd there was a much more vicious attack, signed 'Lynx': he was a foe and not a friend to academic teaching, the discovery of chloroform was a happy go lucky experiment, he was against a classical education, he was unpunctual. Simpson reacted with a brief note to say that he disdained to answer anonymous criticism. The *Courant*, obviously against Simpson, gave a forecast of the result with three of the Curators in his favour and four (including the three University members) against him.

The rising tide of opposition and calumny distressed Simpson but he was not one to acknowledge defeat. His worry and pre-occupation is shown in many letters and in countless rough drafts prepared in answer to his critics. He tried to find out from Gibson Craig what Syme had written in his fateful letter but received a terse reply: 'I cannot give you Syme's letter because considering it was not worth preserving I destroyed it'. He consulted with his lawyers about the Rev. Blackie's letter and about the slanders in the local newspapers. He was advised that if he brought a case for libel against the authors he would succeed. The editor refused to divulge the identity of 'Lynx' and so this particular action could not be pursued.

Just before the appointed date of the election Simpson wrote to the Curators: [220]

As I am informed through one of the Curators that a document has been circulated among them, in it, my religious and moral character is defamed, in order to advance the chances of another candidate for the Principalship—and also another document signed by several of my colleagues, in it they have expressed an opinion that my election would not be advantageous for the University. I have to demand in common fairness that before an election takes place I be allowed an opportunity of hearing and answering openly the charges brought against me. This I am ready and prepared to do.

Late in June William Chambers the Lord Provost, Chairman of the Curators, was on holiday. He had already heard of charges against Simpson, to whom he was giving support, and in some alarm he wrote to Dr Alexander Wood: [221]

. . . he is accused of a want of punctuality and deficiency of business habits—so much so that he could drift into confusion. I have written to Sir James asking if he will give up all that part of his professional practice which would interfere with his duties.

Chambers was anxious to help Simpson and was uninfluenced by the kind of criticism which Blackie had advanced. Simpson replied to the Lord Provost's letter: [222]

In answer to your Lordship's note allow me to state that if elected to the Principalship I shall certainly devote myself thoroughly to the duties of office and perform them, I trust, in a way that will reflect credit upon the University and upon the Curators. I shall not allow my professional work to interfere with the full and conscientious discharge of the paramount duties of the Principalship.

I have now been twenty-eight years a Professor, I have never been absent from my class-room when it was possible at all to be there.

Although much influential support was being diverted to Grant the bulk of the medical profession remained faithful and did their best to counteract the effect of the memorial from the 12 professors. At the last minute the Edinburgh graduates collected 800 signatures to a memorial in support of Simpson. Simpson himself redoubled his efforts and in the last days he replied to every criticism advanced against him. There is a draft of a letter in his own hand and this may have been circulated in his support by the two Colleges: [223]

We the undersigned, the Presidents and Fellows of the College of Physicians and Surgeons . . . having heard that an attempt is being made to prevent Sir James Simpson Bart from being appointed Principal . . . on the grounds that he is not in good terms with, and that his appointment would be unpopular to, his Professional Brethren . . . we feel it an act of justice to Sir James to testify that we believe that there are few men who have done so much good, and thereby created so much jealousy, who have had fewer quarrels and that at this moment we believe him to be at least as popular with every member of the Profession as any Professor in the University.

We know few men of greater urbanity, more real philanthropy, more hospitality or with more real and unaffected kindness than Sir James.

Exhausted and often ill Simpson drafted the answers to each item brought against him in the anonymous attacks in the Edinburgh press. He had been accused of denigrating the value of a classical education, to most Victorian educationalists a terrible heresy. A year or two previously he had given a public lecture at Granton in which he expressed a strong, and quite justifiable, opinion that there was too much emphasis on Latin and Greek at school and university and that it would be better to teach the modern languages. Once more he was ahead of his time but when he said 'classical students were uninformed and often ignorant of their own 'ignorance' this was intolerable to many. He had good reason to be hurt at the criticism that he was 'not fitted to show hospitality to distinguished scientific visitors to Edinburgh': in the previous 20 years he had probably entertained more distinguished strangers than all the other professors put together. To the objection that many of the Senate would not co-operate with him as Principal he answered that there were only three or four and these were the men who had opposed him originally when he became Professor in 1840. That he had 'done his utmost to suppress all pursuits of genuine philosophical acquirements' and that his intellectual achievements were negligible seemed to him scarcely to require an answer. He asked to be given the opportunity of defending his moral and religious character for this was the criticism which hurt most of all.[224]

It was all of no avail for Grant was elected Principal on July 6th. Four of the Curators, including the three University members, voted for Grant while three City members voted for Simpson. The crucial vote was Black's and there was much feeling in Edinburgh that he was instrumental in losing Simpson the Principalship. Simpson was exhausted and depressed when he heard the news. He was, however, a good loser and took the defeat with resignation. Despite everything he refused to bring legal action against his detractors or to speak against them in public. As things turned out Grant proved an able Principal, holding the office until 1884; for Simpson the sands were running out and he had only two years to live.

The popularity of Simpson was widespread and in many quarters his rejection was greatly deplored. In retrospect it is clear that the professorial faction headed by Syme and Christison won the day. As a close second came the influence of those such as Blackie who had cast doubts on Simpson's moral character and who had taken exception to the evangelistic activities in which he had indulged. Perhaps the only valid criticisms of Simpson were for his lack of business acumen, his unpunctuality and the possibility that past quarrels might have made it difficult for him to have conducted the business of the Senate effectively.

In a masterly piece of understatement Duns dismisses the affair with the sentence: 'But, indeed, there was on both sides not a little of the busybodyism which, on such occasions, often works much mischief among friends'. This was written in 1873 and perhaps Duns was wise not to tell all he knew, for most of the protagonists were still living. Simpson's champions thought otherwise and no sooner was the result announced than they conducted an inquisition. Even before the election they had begun to investigate the rumours and the alleged libels. By October three friends, Dr Alexander Wood, Mr Pender and Mr McKie, reported to Simpson and had printed the results of their investigations on the conduct of the election. They had summoned those whom they thought guilty of slander or sharp practice to a court of enquiry and, rather surprisingly, most obeyed the summons quite meekly! First they tried to get the details of Syme's letter but already he had refused to speak and no one else was inclined to remember what had been read out to the Curators. Then they went into the circumstances of the publicity afforded to the Rev. Blackie's letter to Fyfe. There seems little doubt but that it had all been cunningly organised so that as many people saw the letter as possible. The Rev. Blackie apologised to Simpson and said rather lamely that his words had been misconstrued. Professor Fraser apologised and said he thought the letter was open to everyone to read. Professor Christison apologised and said he did not at the time see anything libellous in the letter but he admitted that he had at once shown it to a friend of Simpson's in the hope that it would encourage him to retire gracefully. No one explained why the Rev. Blackie's son had gone to Professor Fraser's house. Professor Muirhead, who was less directly involved, was also summoned before the tribunal but he wrote that he would 'not be interviewed by a self-elected inquisitional triumvirate'. Simpson's friends were perhaps satisfied that they had cleared his name and presumably their printed report had some private circulation. No note was taken of it in the press, directly or indirectly, and by the time it appeared Simpson had already decided to go no further in the matter or to take legal action. He had conducted himself honourably and he was exonerated from blame concerning the use he made of the Bombay telegram.

A large question mark hangs over Syme's behaviour. It may be charitable to suggest that he was actuated by a firm belief that Simpson would have been a bad choice. On matters of principle Syme never wavered but acted according to his conscience. Perhaps his public statement in the Memorial from the 12 professors can be condoned, but there is more than a suspicion that he exceeded the bounds of fairness, or even morality, when he wrote privately to the Curators.

Shattering although the loss of the Principalship was to Simpson, there was compensation in the many honours by which the nation showed their appreciation of his work and merit. In January 1866 he was awarded a baronetcy. He had been offered a title on two previous occasions and this time he was persuaded by his friends to accept. Congratulations came from the humble and the great. The medical world thought such recognition long overdue and preparations were made for a banquet in his honour, but the festivities were cancelled when a few days after the baronetcy was announced his eldest son died. David Simpson qualified as a doctor in 1863 and had shown great promise. As assistant to his father he had begun to appear as the natural successor to the Chair of Obstetrics. Simpson was overwhelmed by his loss and his depression was accentuated when a month later his daughter, Jessie, a chronic invalid, died also. Soon, however, he showed his remarkable resilience and in an attempt to forget his tribulations threw himself with energy into his professional work and all his outside interests.[225]

Both Syme and Simpson received many honorary degrees from universities at home and abroad and were given innumerable foreign decorations. It is a little surprising that Syme was not knighted, not only for his professional achievements but also for the part he had played in furthering the cause of medical education and, in particular, for his long service to the General Medical Council. He may have refused such recognition but there were many who thought that he was neglected.

Perhaps it was a little tactless to honour the two professors at the same ceremony but when the British Medical Association met in Dublin this happened. Both were given honorary doctorates and the President, Dr Stokes, introduced the two distinguished recipients. That evening there was a dinner to celebrate the occasion and Simpson had the place of honour by the President. After the event he wrote to a friend with a certain amount of satisfaction: [226]

> In all meetings and places I had the seat of honour thrust upon me which involved a great deal of speaking. We had a great dinner of nearly 500 doctors. I was placed at the side of the President (Dr Stokes) and to drink his health. While I spoke —Mr Syme who sat opposite and down did look very unhappy as the audience cheered wildly.

While Syme was now greatly respected for his contributions to surgery and to medical education and now largely forgiven for what appeared to some as arrogant and uncompromising behaviour, it was Simpson who was greeted with spontaneous enthusiasm wherever he went. Both were now the elder statesmen of the profession and were called on to deliver numerous addresses at conferences and on special occasions. It fell to Syme to deliver the annual address on surgery at the British Medical Association at Leamington in 1865. It was a rather regrettable performance although it conformed to many such addresses. The subject was the progress of surgery but it really turned out to be the progress of Syme. Almost every contribution he had made was catalogued and there was little reference to the work of others. As already recorded he took the opportunity once more of attacking Lizars in a vehement manner. There was an attack on Simpson also and the medical press were quick to notice that Syme denied his colleague any credit for his contribution to medicine: 'the mind of the Professor is in a most peculiar state of etherisation as to the discovery of chloroform—a state which also renders him quite insensible to the use of pins and needles for certain surgical purposes'. It was rather sad that with the opportunity offered on such an occasion Syme seemed incapable of expressing generosity towards others, nor had the facility to evaluate new ideas or to attempt some forecast of the future of surgery. Harshly although Syme might be criticised for such egoism there are indications that his true character was misrepresented by his public utterances. In 1866 he presided at a dinner of the Edinburgh University Club in London. Grudgingly the *Lancet* reported the deep regard of his friends: [227]

> For it is a most creditable peculiarity of Mr Syme to enjoy to a very high degree the esteem, we had almost said the affection, of his pupils. . . . This remark may be scarcely intelligible to those who are only familiar with the polemical aspects of Mr Syme's character. . . . All the style of the man flashed upon them as if only yesterday they had been his pupils.

Up to 1869 Syme had enjoyed good health but from the photographs of this period it is apparent that he had begun to age markedly. On April 10th while in his carriage on the way to his consulting room he had a stroke. He developed a left sided paralysis but in a few days there was a rapid recovery. By the summer he felt that he should resign his professorship and there was a spontaneous expression throughout the country of respect and gratitude for his long service. Many felt that the Government should now award him a knighthood but this was not to be. His friends and his former students inaugurated a fund to provide tangible expressions of their esteem in the form of a marble bust and a fellowship to be awarded in his name.

The appointment of his successor created much interest and Bell, Spence, Heron Watson and Lister were the fancied candidates. Syme exerted all the influence he could to appoint his son-in-law, who was undoubtedly the right choice. There were the usual accusations of nepotism from some quarters and there was a strong proposal to abolish the Chair altogether. Spence was at the time President of the College of Surgeons and already held a Chair of Surgery. He had powerful support but much was made of a recent incident in the Infirmary when Spence, who was against the antiseptic doctrine, had attributed a fatal post-operative result to the use of cat-gut and had victimised Syme's house-surgeon Edward Laurie, because he had contradicted Spence's account of the case. It must have given Syme great satisfaction to see Lister take up his work; he attended the new professor's inaugural address and gave all the support possible to establish him in his new position.[228]

Syme was now content to withdraw from public life and his clinical contributions ceased except for his brief references to his experience of the antiseptic method. There were a few terse and characteristic letters to the press on the subject of medical education, which revealed that he still retained an active interest in affairs and had not lost his aggressive spirit. On May 26th 1870 he suffered a second and more severe stroke which rendered him partially paralysed and speechless. Cared for by his old friends Brown and Peddie, he suffered a lingering decline and died at Millbank on June 26th.

In 1868 Simpson was called upon once more to address the new medical graduates. He exhorted them to unremitting study and warned them of the pitfalls before them. In extolling the value of the new techniques such as microscopy, ophthalmoscopy and laryngoscopy he encouraged them to seek out further means of diagnosis and said:[229]

Possibly even, by the concentration of electrical or other lights, we may yet render many parts of the body, if not the whole body, sufficiently diaphanous for the inspection of the practised eye of the physician and surgeon.

Some enthusiasts have regarded this as a forecast of the discovery of X-ray examination and at least it shows how Simpson was constantly seeking new ways of improving the art of diagnosis.

There were many other equally inspiring addresses, particularly to wider audiences on matters of public health. He had new ideas on the eradication of smallpox, on population problems and on housing. His originality is seen when he elaborated on the disposal of sewage, deploring the enormous loss of fertilisers by pouring waste products into the sea. To the end of life he kept abreast of all scientific thought and development.

All this time he was to be seen regularly at meetings of the societies in Edinburgh and at conferences all over the country. But overwork, lack of sleep, hurried meals and exhausting journeys were taking their toll. Despite his apparently inexhaustible physical reserves his work began to be interrupted by periods of illness. He was subject to attacks of migraine and sciatica and was often prostrated by such illnesses. For years he had allowed himself only a few hours of sleep but now he had become the victim of insomnia. He experimented with the new drug chloral and there were rumours that he over-dosed himself. Finally he began to suffer distressing anginal attacks and had to resort to inhalation of his own chloroform for relief. There were periods of mental depression related to his domestic sorrows and to his exhausting conflicts. Usually these attacks were short-lived and his natural optimism and ebullience rose above the shadows. Although increasingly crippled by heart disease, so that to climb a staircase became almost impossible, he did not let up but continued to work at the same tempo as of old. Early in 1870 he had to travel repeatedly to London to give evidence in a divorce case and thereafter, exhausted mentally and physically, he answered an urgent summons to Perth to manage a difficult obstetrical case. When he returned he took to his bed and there was a progressive deterioration in his con-

dition. Ill although he was he carried on his medical writing
and his archaeological studies. His last letters to the journals
were to defend himself against the accusations of Dr Bigelow
of New York. Simpson had received the Freedom of the City
of Edinburgh in 1869, he made an impromptu speech and
in some of the reports it seemed that he had claimed to be the
discoverer of general anaesthesia. Dr Bigelow wrote long
and angry letters to substantiate the claims of the Americans
in introducing ether anaesthesia. Simpson wrote even longer
letters denying that he had suggested that he had done more
than to introduce chloroform and to establish general anaesthesia in childbirth. For two months he lay in his house in
Queen Street, often wracked by severe pain. His mind was as
active as ever and he strove to complete his work on hospitalism. He expressed the hope that 'some good man will take it
up'. When Simpson died his pupil Lawson Tait was given
all the statistics and the task of carrying on the fight and
in time he did publish a pamphlet.[230]

Simpson knew he would not recover. He examined his beliefs, aided by Dr Duns who, it would seem, had some satisfaction in supporting the troubled and the repentant on his
death bed. There was love and comfort from all his family and
his last care was to ensure that they were provided for and
that his younger children would be able to continue their
education and upbringing to the best advantage. The course
of his illness was followed in detail by the public and there
was a cloud over the land when it was known that he could
not recover. Surrounded by his family he died on May 6th and
his last words were spoken to his beloved brother Sandy who,
with the others, had so encouraged and supported him
throughout his remarkable life.[231]

CHAPTER 12

Contemporary Eulogy and a Retrospective Judgement

'ONE of our greatest men has passed from amongst us; Simpson is dead!' was the announcement in the *Medical Times and Gazette*. The medical journals had long and adulatory obituaries and the national dailies carried a full coverage of his life and work. At home and abroad Simpson had become a figure of great eminence and to the lay public his greatest fame was for his discovery of chloroform. While in Edinburgh the general feeling of sorrow was more intense and personal, the sense of loss was almost equalled in London. A group of his friends, including Sir William Fergusson, Dr Priestley and Mr Spencer Wells, made approaches to the Dean of Westminster so that Simpson might be given a state funeral in the Abbey. Watt Black, his old pupil, wrote to Walter Simpson: [232]

I hope you will not make any objection to the Westminster Abbey proposal. All seem enthusiastic about it here. You would have a procession in Edinburgh to the Station instead of to Warriston:

I suppose there never was an instance before of a Scotchman being brought up from Scotland to Westminster Abbey.

Already, however, preparations were in hand for an appropriate and elaborate ceremony in Edinburgh. The family preferred that he should be buried in Warriston cemetery where in 1841, on the death of his first child, he had purchased a plot; already three of his children lay there. When the Westminster proposal was rejected Jonathan Hutchison wrote 'I believe in future years, it will be a matter of universal regret that circumstances have prevented the realisation of the proposal which has just been put aside'. The proposal was spontaneous and unique and shows the exceptional regard in which Simpson was held.

The scenes at the funeral were recorded in great detail and it had to be admitted that there had been nothing like it since the death of Thomas Chalmers, the eminent churchman. On May 13th a huge crowd gathered in Queen Street and spilled into the side streets. Every window and even the roof tops were crammed with spectators along the route to Warriston. There was a service in the house attended by the family and by close friends such as Dr Alexander Wood, Mr Pender of Manchester and the young Lawson Tait from Wakefield. Meanwhile a great procession was being marshalled. Representatives of the University, the Colleges and the various societies gathered in their respective halls and then marched to Queen Street in their academic dress. The City Council attended with its full regalia. Every civic, scientific and literary body of importance was represented, from the Town Council of Bathgate to the Granton Literary Society. It was quite a task to create some kind of order in this unprecedented public and private demonstration but there was only an hour's delay before the procession moved off. The funeral car was 'a stately catafalque constructed specially for the occasion by Messrs Croall in the style of an old Roman bier'. It was drawn by six fine Belgian horses and driven by three postillions. That afternoon everything stopped in Edinburgh while the bells of St Giles and other churches tolled. It was estimated that some 80,000 people lined the streets and that 2,000 took part in the official procession. The tribute was genuine for as the cortège wound its way down towards Leith 'the hushed solemnity of the dense crowd of spectators through which it moved was most impressive. Tears streamed down many cheeks, and frequently sobs, as from hearts bearing a deep personal sorrow, fell on the ear'. At Canonmills a group of waifs and strays, from a home in which Simpson had been interested, were gathered to bid farewell to their benefactor. Late in the afternoon, in the failing sunshine, Simpson was buried where he had wished to be, with the prospect to the south of the Castle Rock, the spires and turrets from St Giles to Holyrood, the high tenements of the High Street and the crouching mass of Arthur's Seat.[233]

Letters of condolence came to the family from all ranks of society, from the Queen to the humblest patient. Sermons were preached in the Edinburgh churches and medical societies throughout the world suspended their business to indulge in lengthy tributes. In some quarters there were waves of almost excessive emotion, either to exaggerate his merits as an evangelical preacher or to accord him an excessive credit in the development of anaesthesia. There was an outburst of laudatory and sentimental pamphlets and of indifferent poems. The *British Medical Journal* struck a cautious note: 'The public has accorded him a greater sphere of merit than was his due—he appeared to yield a little to the temptation of receiving praises . . . offered in some degree of error'.

Simpson had died in harness at the peak of his reputation and it was not surprising that plans were at once made for a memorial. A subscription list was opened and the response was immediate, including £200 from Duncan Flockhart Ltd who owed to Simpson a highly profitable trade in chloroform. The main project was the erection of a statue in Princes Street. This was sculptured by William Brodie and cast in bronze in London. There were some vicissitudes, when it was unshipped at Leith an arm came off, but in 1873 it was unveiled by Lady Galloway before a distinguished gathering, with due ceremony and oratory. In London his memory was perpetuated by the placing of a fine portrait medallion in Westminster Abbey, beside the memorials to other great British doctors and scientists. As a further tribute a new maternity hospital in Edinburgh was named after him, but some thought this an unsuitable tribute in considering his views on hospital construction.[234]

The baronetcy passed to the second son, Walter. He had studied Law in Cambridge and Edinburgh but practised his profession only sporadically. He achieved some fame as 'Athelred', the friend of Robert Louis Stevenson, his contemporary as a law student in Edinburgh. He frequently travelled with the writer and was his companion on the canoe trip immortalised in *An Inland Voyage*. Stevenson was the eccentric on these excursions, in dress as well as habits, while Walter Simpson acted as a respectable foil when there were crises in hotels or elsewhere. He had the capacity for 'eloquent silences' while Stevenson held forth far into the night. The second baronet lived the life of a country squire and his one contribution to literature was quite a popular work *The Art of Golf*. In 1898 Sir Walter died and was succeeded by his son James whose career was short and undistinguished. On the death of James the baronetcy became void but there are direct descendants of the family through his daughter. Of Simpson's other surviving children Eve lived until 1919. She was a lady of great character and an author of some merit. In addition to the biography of her father she wrote two or three books on R. L. Stevenson. Although these are rather chatty and light they hardly deserve a recent criticism as 'tiresomely inadequate', for because of Walter's friendship she was in a position to fill in interesting details of Stevenson's early life in Edinburgh. Another son William seems to have been rather a failure; he was an eccentric painter who was fond of absinthe in which he indulged with his bull-terrier which had similar tastes! Alexander Magnus Simpson, the godson of Simpson's friend Magnus Retzius, qualified in medicine but did not have a particularly notable career.[235]

Simpson's brother Alexander had several children and from this branch of the family there are many to whom the genius and ability of Simpson's forbears were transmitted. Of this family Alexander Russel Simpson (1835–1919) qualified in medicine. He acted as assistant to his uncle between 1860 and 1870 and succeeded him in the Chair of Obstetrics. Few professors had such an inauspicious start for the students and others were in complete opposition to his election. The main rival was Matthews Duncan who by 1870 had acquired a great reputation, although now an antagonist to Simpson, and was thought to be the certain choice. To some the election of Alexander Simpson was seen as a disgraceful example of family influence exerted, in this instance, beyond the grave! His introductory lecture was a shambles and it was a full five minutes before the catcalls and the showers of missiles subsided and he was allowed to proceed. Soon, however, he was accepted and he proved a worthy successor to his more famous uncle.[236]

Lady Simpson survived her husband for only a month. There is evidence of her complete faithfulness and love for her husband in the few letters between them which survive after the romantic courtship in 1839. Her unfailing devotion to her family and her management of a household subjected to the tempestuous habits and extravagant hospitality of her partner must place her high in the list of innumerable, long-suffering doctors' wives, who contribute so much, if indirectly, to medical progress. The loss of so many of her children took a heavy toll of her physical, and perhaps mental, health and in her later years it seems that she suffered frequent depressive illnesses which added to her husband's domestic trials.[237]

When Syme died on June 20th the news was not unexpected for he had been ill for some months. There had already been full tributes to his work and character in the demonstrations of affection and respect accorded on his retiral from the professorship. The notices of his death were lavish in their praises but there was not quite the same sense of public loss as was evinced so overwhelmingly when Simpson died. It was in character that his funeral was private and that there was none of the civic pomp which attended Simpson's obsequies. He was buried in the family vault in the small sunk graveyard lying to the east of St John's episcopal church, of which he had been a faithful member. Christison, Peddie, Brown and Principal Grant represented the University and of his firm friends and pupils there came Sharpey from London and Dobie from Chester.[238]

His second wife had died a year previously and one son and three daughters survived. James Syme, the younger, lived on at Millbank until about 1880 but no record can be traced of his career or if he married. Agnes, the wife of Joseph Lister, died in 1893. Her sister Lucy was unmarried and went to care for Lister in his declining years. Paterson mentions also a third daughter by Syme's second wife who married a Major Burn; no direct descendants through this union have been traced. The tangible memorials of Syme are the marble busts by Brodie in the Royal Infirmary and in the University, various portraits and the surgical fellowship still

244

awarded in Edinburgh in his name.[239]

It remains to make some final assessment of the character and achievement of these two men. Already striking contrasts must be apparent and something more may be learned by quoting the opinions of their contemporaries.

It has been shown that Syme appeared to all but his personal friends as somewhat harsh, uncompromising and quarrelsome but an anonymous correspondent in *The Scotsman* in 1870 wrote: 'Many have judged him severely, have thought him harsh and of a hasty temper but we who knew him feel how much he has been wronged.' All his obituarists were at pains to make the same qualifications. He was credited with 'uncompromising truthfulness', a quality so pronounced that if he thought anyone was wrong in his surgical beliefs, that man was a knave. If he considered that criticism was just then he could not conceal his feelings; 'he lacked the varnish which conceals the sting without depriving it of venom'. It is often the case that a strict disciplinarian gains respect and even affection; these were given to Syme by almost all his colleagues and his pupils.

John Brown and Joseph Lister pronounced what may be the true verdicts on his character. Both were reliable judges and both knew Syme intimately. Brown is shown by his writings as one of the most perceptive of men and his assessment clearly comes from the heart. A letter from Brown to Lister in 1869, when Syme was recovering from his first stroke, is simple and revealing; 'Mr Syme is wonderfully well and so good and gentle and considerate. I don't think I ever knew a better human being'. In all his comments Brown brings out a basic simplicity, integrity and humanity in Syme's character, summing up in classical panegyric, 'Verax, Capax, Perspicax, Sagax, Efficax, Tenax'.[240]

Lister's opinion is of equal significance for he was completely honest and, from his Quaker origins, a sensitive judge of his fellow men. He wrote in *The Scotsman* of June 28th: [241]

The most prominent feature of Mr Syme's character was uncompromising truthfulness; and with the love of what was true and noble was combined, in a corresponding measure, the detestation of what he believed to be counterfeit and base. As he expressed his sentiments with the utmost candour, he not infrequently gave personal offence, though, in the majority of cases, this was only transient. But whatever may have been thought of his free speaking by some individuals, the profession and the world at large owe him an incalculable debt of gratitude for the noble stand he was at all times ready to make against meanness and falsehood. . . .

The hostility which he excited in a few was greatly out-weighed by the friendship he inspired in the many. Rarely is it granted to any one to attach to himself the enduring love and admiration of so large a number of his fellow-men. This was due not only to his perfect genuineness of character, which could not fail to gain respect even from those who differed from him, but also to another quality, as essential as truth-fulness to a good surgeon—a most warm heart, a true love for his fellow creatures, and a general appreciation of sterling merit in whatever form it might present itself. Mr Syme, in short, besides being a surgical genius of the highest order, was a perfect gentleman, and a good, as well as a great man.

This generous tribute can be balanced against the less favourable comments during and after Syme's life time. We see him as one whose basic shyness was often evinced by a truculent attitude towards his fellows. He lacked tact and probably he lacked a sense of humour. There could be no compromise or deviation from the principles in which he believed. He himself had some awareness of his faults, for when he spoke at the dinner given in his honour before he went to London he was reported to have said 'he had often expressed opinions when silence would have been more con-ducive to his own quiet and professional advancement . . . he had never entered into any contention unless necessary to vindicate some principle which he thought it his duty to maintain'.

He was outstanding in a period of unparalleled progress in surgery and he was seen by his contemporaries as the guiding force, pronouncing judgement on all that was new and holding fast to old doctrines which he believed well proven. His work on joint diseases and aneurysms and his original method of amputation at the ankle joint were accepted by his fellows as his most important contributions to surgery. His text-books and his unique method of clinical teaching were held to be of even more importance, for all his teaching had a great influence far beyond the Edinburgh school. It was perhaps apt that one commentator described him as the Wellington rather than the Napoleon of surgery.

The contemporary opinions of Simpson were expressed very fully when he died. It was admitted that there were complexities in his make-up: 'The emotional in his nature was easily aroused and deeply felt, enhancing all his pleasure and augmenting all his pains'. It was clear to all that Simpson had felt deeply for his fellow men and women and that he had been blessed with a magnetic personality through which he transmitted to his patients an exceptional degree of confidence. It was written of him that no man was ever more greatly loved, that he was humble-minded, kind-hearted and benevolent to a fault. He was said to have preserved a coolness of temper even in the most trying circumstances but if he did become deeply involved in a quarrel and was hasty or ungenerous he was ready to forgive and forget. His susceptibility to new ideas was thought to be such that sometimes he got carried away and showed a lack of judgement. At his death there were many who deplored his religious teaching and he himself seemed to have realised that he had entered this field inadequately prepared. His life was measured against his humble origin, his intense ambition and his determination to aid mankind by the advancement of medical science. His rise to fame undoubtedly gave him great satisfaction but behind all this there was recognised a sense of humility fostered by his simple but firm religious beliefs.

At the time of Simpson's death there was a popular view that his place in history would be assured mainly by his work on anaesthesia. His contributions to obstetrics and gynaecology, however, were well established and his influence as a teacher in these subjects was accepted as unique. Hospitalism was still under review and the significance of his views on this subject are more readily evaluated today than was possible in 1870. One correspondent observed: 'His reputation will ripen with the years, jealousies will be forgotten and antagonisms will be merged'. There were few exceptions to the general feeling in 1870 that the world had lost a genius.

The achievement of these two men may be measured by their influence on their own time and by considering to what extent their ideas are pertinent today. In an age of rapid development in all the sciences they were complementary to each other. Syme's cautious and conservative outlook was needed to counteract the over-enthusiastic and sometimes reckless applications of new ideas and inventions. Simpson with his original and critical mind was needed equally to exploit what was new for the benefit of mankind.

Syme entered his career when the repertoire of the surgeon was restricted and when surgery had no scientific background. When he died the field had widened remarkably and with the benefits of general anaesthesia and of the understanding of wound infection, the surgeon was no longer a crude technician. To the main-stream of surgery he contributed much even although the particular techniques he devised scarcely survive today. His ingenious amputation at the ankle-joint is now rarely employed: his excision of major joints for tuberculosis are now seldom required and his stricture operation is of no importance. But all such operations and his radical approach to tumours and aneurysms were important in their time and from them was built up much of modern surgical technique. In his day he had great authority, not only in Edinburgh but throughout the world, by his teaching to students and by his writings. He exerted an influence at least equal to that of Liston, Fergusson, Brodie and other surgical giants of the time. It was his ambition to be a leader in surgery and this he undoubtedly achieved. Further, by the introduction of his method of clinical instruction and by his active participation in the reform of medical training and practice he greatly influenced teaching and the status of the doctor in the British Isles.

Simpson found obstetrics confused and ill-taught. If he had done nothing else he would be remembered for his establishment of this specialty on sound principles and in equality with medicine and surgery. This he did by his able teaching to his students, by his research and by the development of countless new techniques. There was scarcely any aspect of obstetrical science on which he did not write and if he demolished false conceptions he replaced them with well proven doctrines. In his life time he was accepted as the leader in obstetrics. He may be seen also as the founder of gynaecology as a separate specialty. By his exploitation of new methods of diagnosis he brought order into this field: against great opposition he established the use of the uterine sound, the exploring needle and the speculum. It was equally important that he overcame the strong element of prudery of the age, on account of which the obstetricians and gynaecologists were restricted, not only in the use of essential diagnostic techniques, but also in asking questions necessary for the understanding of their cases.[242]

Simpson's range of activity was wide and by his work on acupressure, on hospital infection and on statistics he influenced surgical progress markedly. In medicine his writings against homoeopathy did much towards the establishment of rational therapy. His contributions to anaesthesia went far beyond the introduction of chloroform for it was his successful campaign to persuade others to use general anaesthesia, both in midwifery and surgery, which stamped him as a true benefactor.

Each therefore has an important place in the history of medicine. The influence of Syme is not perhaps carried onwards so directly as that of Simpson; it may be said that in surgery he played an important part in the evolution and passed on the torch to others. The debt which is owed to him is not easily calculated but is far from negligible. Simpson with his wider interests and his capacity for looking ahead has left a greater mark. Most of the ideas for which he incurred the most severe criticism survive to this day. Even now the question of giving to all women in labour the relief afforded by skilled anaesthesia is still a subject of concern. Anaesthetists, now united as a specialist body equal with the surgeons, still strive for the perfect agent, as Simpson did, however satisfied he was with chloroform. When Simpson advocated acupressure he expressed the hope that something better would be found than his method of ligation; today surgeons continue this search and diathermy coagulation has been developed as a remarkably effective alternative. His advocacy of metallic sutures is still supported strongly in certain branches of surgery. At the beginning of the 1939 war the surgeons, encouraged by the teaching of Trueta from his experience in the Spanish Civil War, had to look afresh at the simple doctrines so clearly expounded by Simpson on the management of wounds—relief of tension, clearance of dead tissues, insistence on haemostasis and avoidance of tight sutures.

But most of all it is to Simpson's views on hospitals to which we may turn profitably today. Although fatalities from sepsis are now rare, a high morbidity from wound infection in hospital remains a cause of suffering and is an economic disaster. These things are not yet solved despite all the refinements of bacteriological technique and antibiotic therapy. Such problems are directly associated with the simple fact which Simpson so often stressed, that patients should not be crowded together in open wards. Simpson had the conviction that hospitals should not be massive palaces built to last a century or more and he advocated simple prefabricated structures which could be replaced cheaply and quickly according to varying needs. By the failure to appreciate his reasoning we have in this country a legacy of almost indestructible Victorian monuments, ill-planned to prevent infection, often ill-sited and always difficult and expensive to adapt to the changing needs of medical science. The money devoted to their maintenance and conversion leaves little to spare for their immediate substitution by simpler, safer and more economic units. This is only one of the lessons which we may learn from Simpson, who in so many things was ahead of his time.

With the passing of a hundred years Simpson emerges as the more vivid and the more attractive character and is the greater of the two men. Admittedly his image is transmitted to us so freshly in his own writings, in the memoirs of his family and in contemporary records of all kinds. He sought the limelight and it is significant that he did not destroy his letters and papers but that they survive for posterity. Syme was more reticent and although the impact of his different personality is revealed by some, the information available to us concerning his life is much less in quantity. Both were great men and take an honoured place in history for their humanity, industry and contribution to the progress of medical science.

Some may consider that by their intrigues and personal

rivalry both Simpson and Syme are reduced in stature. This aspect of their lives must be seen in its true context and should not be over-stressed. It has been said 'controversy, particularly acrimonious controversy, is one of the privileges of a civilised life' and certainly this was true of the Victorian period.

We may halt for a moment on the pavement of the East End of Princes Street and look upwards at Simpson's statue and then to Syme's grave nearby and remember these two remarkable Scotsmen, forgetting the quarrels but marvelling that despite all trials and difficulties they achieved so much.

Biographical Sources

JAMES SYME

The only full biography is by Robert Paterson, *Memorials of the Life of James Syme,* published in 1874 in Edinburgh by Edmonston and Douglas (*see* Preface). There are a few shorter accounts including the following:

BROWN, J. N. E. (1941). Syme and his son-in-law. *Ann. med. Hist.,* 3, 18.

GRAHAM, J. (1954). James Syme 1799–1870. *Br. J. plast. Surg.,* 7, 1.

MACLEAN, D. (1898). Personal reminiscences of Syme. *Med. Age,* 61, 34.

PEDDIE, A. (1890). *Dr John Brown: his Life and Work. With Narrative Sketches of James Syme.* (Pamphlet printed in Edinburgh.)

PEMBERTON, O. (1894). James Syme. (Bradshaw Lecture at the Royal College of Surgeons of England.) *Lancet,* 2, 1399.

There is information about Syme in the biographies of Joseph Lister and in the writings of contemporaries such as Dr John Brown and Professor Christison.

I have failed to trace any large collection of letters or other documents relating to Syme. Paterson must have had access to such letters as survived after 1870, those for example between Syme and Sharpey, and some of these are quoted. There are a few letters written by Syme in the Edinburgh University Library along with his diplomas from foreign universities and medical societies, various pamphlets and lecture notes taken by his students. Some letters are in the Royal College of Surgeons of Edinburgh and in the Lister Collection in the Royal College of Surgeons of England.

JAMES SIMPSON

Three biographies have been used freely. The most detailed is that by the Rev. John Duns, *Memoir of Sir James Y. Simpson* published by Edmonston and Douglas in Edinburgh in 1873. Two shorter accounts are Eve Simpson's *Sir James Y. Simpson* published by Scribner, New York in 1896 in the 'Famous Scots' series and Dr Gordon Lang's *Sir James Young Simpson and Chloroform* (1811–1870) published by Unwin, London in 1897 in the 'Masters of Medicine' series. Both of these owe much to Duns. (*See* Preface.)

There are many shorter accounts of Simpson's life. Those which appeared soon after his death emphasise his evangelical activities. The Rev. Charles Bullock, for example, gives a rather sanctimonious essay entitled *The Man of Science, The Man of God*. There is a similar sketch by M. F. Barbour in *Golden Vials Filled*. *James Young Simpson, Twenty Years and Their Lessons*, reprinted from the *Scots Observer* of 1891 for private circulation, is an anonymous assessment of Simpson's character and a defence against the slanders not infrequently brought against him.

On the centenary of Simpson's birth in 1911 a whole number of the *Edinburgh Medical Journal* (vol. 6, p. 482) was devoted to his commemoration. The contributions by Eve Simpson and by Professor Sir Alexander Simpson are noteworthy. In 1947, on the centenary of the discovery of the use of chloroform, a further series of commemorative articles appeared in the same journal.

The Royal College of Obstetricians and Gynaecologists inaugurated an annual oration in Simpson's memory in 1961 (endowed by Mr V. B. Green-Armytage). A Simpson memorial lecture was instituted in Edinburgh in 1965. The list of these orations is appended and some are noted as useful or original sources in the individual chapter references.

R.C.O.G. ORATIONS

1961. MILLER, D., James Y. Simpson—clarum et venerabile nomen gentibus (Lucan). (A name illustrious and revered by nations.) *J. Obstet. Gynaec. Br. Commonw.* (1962). *69*, 142–150.

1962. WILLIAMS, L., Simpson, the teacher and those that follow him. *J. Obstet. Gynaec. Br. Commonw.* (1963). *70*, 167–172.

1963. MOIR, J. C., Sir J. Y. Simpson: his impact and influence. *J. Obstet. Gynaec. Br. Commonw.* (1964). *71*, 171–179.

1964. TAYLOR, C. W., Lawson Tait—a grateful pupil of James Young Simpson. *J. Obstet. Gynaec. Br. Commonw.* (1965). *72*, 165–171.

1965. KENNEDY, C. D., Sir James Young Simpson: the splendid ultimate triumph. *J. Obstet. Gynaec. Br. Commonw.* (1966). *73*, 364–371.

1966. ANDERSON, D. F., Ethics, aesthetics and anaesthetics. (Unpublished.)

1967. GUNN, A., James Young Simpson, the complete gynaecologist. *J. Obstet. Gynaec. Br. Commonw.* (1968). *75*, 249–263.

1968. COSBIE, W. G. Simpson and some Canadian contemporaries. (Not yet published.)

SIMPSON MEMORIAL LECTURE

1965. KELLAR, R. J. Sir James Young Simpson—victor dolore. *Jl. R. Coll. Surg. Edinb.* (1966). *12*, 1.

As far as letters and other personal documents are concerned there is an almost embarrassing amount of material. In 1948 the Royal College of Surgeons of Edinburgh was given the custody of a large trunk of papers. There are letters on every conceivable topic, from or to Simpson, and documents which throw light on the more obscure facets of his career, for example, the election for the Principalship of the University. This collection was available to Duns and to Eve Simpson and may have been seen by Lang. While Duns quotes many of the letters he did not use all the information available in these papers, probably because many of the persons involved were still living in 1873. The documents are not, unfortunately, arranged chronologically or in relation to subject matter but it is to be hoped that in time they will be catalogued, representing as they do an invaluable source of information to the medical historian. Where I have quoted from letters or other papers I have used the originals and not Duns' versions which are often out of context and undated.

The College of Surgeons of Edinburgh holds a separate collection of letters. To the best of my knowledge some of those which I quote have not been published previously. Recently Miss Catherine Simpson has presented to the College a batch of letters written between 1858 and 1864 by Simpson to Spencer Wells. These were sent to Sir Alexander Simpson by Wells in

1892. Miss Simpson has allowed me to quote also certain letters concerning the Crimean War which are of exceptional interest.

In the Royal College of Physicians of Edinburgh there is a large collection of material such as personal note-books, bound reprints, lecture drafts and the residue of Simpson's personal library.

I have no doubt that there are other letters and documents scattered throughout the world which I have not traced. In Liverpool I have been fortunate to have ready access in the library of the Medical Institution to a large dossier on the Waldie controversy.

Selected Writings of James Syme

This list includes all Syme's books and monographs and his more important or interesting articles in the journals. He was a prolific writer but it has not been thought necessary to include all the articles and case reports from his pen. Writings referred to in the text are included, in particular those not listed in the chapter references.

1824. Successful case of amputation at the hip joint. *Edinb. med. surg. J.*, *21*, 19.

1825. Remarks on the treatment of incised wounds. *Edinb. med. surg. J.*, *24*, 52.

1826. Cases in which the head of the humerus was successfully excised. *Edinb. med surg. J.*, *26*, 49.

1828. Essay on the nature of inflammation. *Edinb. med. surg. J.*, *30*, 316.

1828. Case of osteo-sarcoma of the lower jaw removed by James Syme Esq. *Edinb. med. surg. J.*, *30*, 286.

1829. Quarterly report of the Edinburgh Surgical Hospital. *Edinb. med. surg. J.*, *32*, 231. (Twelve such reports were continued until 1834 and reveal Syme's surgical practice in the Minto House period.)

1829. Three cases in which the elbow joint was successfully excised, with some general observations on the treatment of caries. *Edinb. med. surg. J.*, *31*, 256.

1829. Superior maxillary bone excised. *Edinb. med. surg. J.*, *32*, 218.

1831. *Treatise on the Excision of Diseased Joints*, Edinburgh.

1831. *Principles of Surgery*, Edinburgh. (First edition in 1831 followed by a fuller text in 1832. Further editions in 1837, 1842 and 1856.)

1835. Clinical reports. *Edinb. med. surg. J.*, *44*, 1. (The first of a long series of reports of Syme's surgical practice in the Royal Infirmary.)

1838. *Diseases of the Rectum,* Edinburgh. (Further editions 1839, 1844 and 1864.)

1839. On the power of the periosteum to form new bone. *Trans. R. Soc. Edinb., 1,* 14.

1841. Surgical cases and observations, *Mon. J. med. Sci., 1,* 1. (Series continued as 'Clinical Lectures' in 1851 until 1855.)

1846. Amputation at the Ankle, *Mon. J. med. Sci., 7,* 81.

1847. On restoration of the upper and lower lips, *Mon. J. med. Sci., 8,* 641.

1847. On the use of ether, *Mon. J. med. Sci., 8,* 72.

1847. Case of axillary aneurysm for which the subclavian artery was tied with success. *Mon. J. med. Sci., 8,* 217.

1848. *Contributions to the Pathology and Practice of Surgery,* Edinburgh.

1848. *On Stricture of the Urethra and Fistula in Perineo,* Edinburgh. (Further editions 1849 and 1855.)

1855. Clinical lectures, *Lancet, 1,* 1. (Series of 22 lectures prepared with the help of Joseph Lister.)

1856. Cases and observations in surgery. *Edinb. med. J., 2,* 1. (Series continued until 1869 under various titles.)

1856. On the radical cure of reducible hernia, *Edinb. med. J., 6,* 865.

1861. *Observations in Clinical Surgery,* Edinburgh.

1862. Case of iliac aneurysm. *Edinb. med. J., 8,* 65.

1864. *Excision of Scapula,* Edinburgh.

1864. Excision of tongue, *Lancet, 1,* 115.

1865. Torsion, ligature and acupressure. *Lancet, 1,* 333.

1865. Ligation of the femoral artery for the 35th time. *Edinb. med. J. 11,* 967.

1867. On the treatment of incised wounds with a view to union by the first intention. *Lancet, 2,* 5.

1868. Illustrations of the antiseptic principle of treatment in surgery. *Bri. med. J., 1,* 1.

Selected Writings of James Simpson

An original intention to provide a full bibliography has proved impracticable. Much of Simpson's writings are duplicated in different journals and the total volume is immense. I have given in this list his more important monographs and articles and include, in particular, those mentioned in the text. Simpson's many articles relating to obstetrics and gynaecology are represented by only a few important or interesting titles. Many of his articles were reprinted for private circulation as pamphlets, sometimes with additional notes. These pamphlets are not always dated and do not always provide the original journal reference. It is, therefore, difficult to catalogue them with any accuracy. They are to be found in some medical libraries such as that of the Liverpool Medical Institution. A separate list is given of Simpson's archaeological studies.

Simpson never completed a full text book on obstetrics and gynaecology but various collected lectures or articles were published before and after his death, both in Great Britain and America. The more important are:

1855. *Simpson's Obstetric Works*, Ed. Priestley, W. O. & Storer, H. R., Edinburgh.

1871. *Selected Obstetrical Works of Sir J. Y. Simpson Bart*, Watt Black, J., Edinburgh.

1871. *Anaesthesia, Hospitalism, Hermaphroditism and a Proposal to Stamp Out Small Pox and other Contagious Diseases*, Ed. Sir W. G. Simpson, Edinburgh.

Papers and Monographs on Medical Subjects

1836. Pathological observations on the diseases of the placenta. *Edinb. med. surg. J.*, *45*, 265.

1838. Contributions to intra-uterine pathology. *Edinb. med. surg. J.*, *50*, 390.

1839. Contributions to intra-uterine pathology. *Edinb. med. surg.*

J., 52, 17.

1839. On the evidence of the occasional contagious propagation of malignant cholera, which is derived from cases of its direct importation into new localities by infected individuals. *Edinb. med. surg. J., 49,* 355.

1843. Contributions to the pathology and treatment of diseases of the uterus. *Mon. J. med. Sci., 3,* 547.

1844. On the alleged infecundity of females born co-twins with males, with some notes on the average proportion of marriages without issue in general society. *Edinb. med. surg. J., 61,* 107.

1844. Memoir on the sex of the child as a cause of difficulty and danger in parturition. *Edinb. med. surg. J., 62,* 387.

1845. Clinical lectures in midwifery and the diseases of women and children. *Mon. J. med. Sci., 5,* 109.

1847. Principles of treatment in placental presentation. *Lancet, 1,* 479.

1847. Notes on the employment of the inhalation of sulphuric ether in the practice of midwifery. *Mon. J. med. Sci., 8,* 721.

1847. Etherisation in surgery. Part I. Its effects, objections to it, etc. *Mon. J. med. Sci., 8,* 145.

1847. Etherisation in surgery. Part II. Proper mode of investigating its effects—statistical propositions and results etc. *Mon. J. med. Sci., 8,* 313.

1847. On a new anaesthetic agent, more efficient than sulphuric ether. *Lancet, 2,* 549.

1847. Cases of the employment of chloroform in midwifery with remarks. *Lancet, 2,* 623.

1847. Anaesthetic and other therapeutical effects of the inhalation of chloroform. *Mon. J. med. Sci., 8,* 415.

1848. Etherisation in surgery. Part III. Does etherisation increase or decrease the mortality attendant upon surgical operations? *Mon. J. med. Sci., 8,* 697.

1848. Report of the Edinburgh Royal Maternity Hospital. *Mon. J. med. Sci., 9,* 328.

1848. On a suction tractor: or new mechanical power as a substitute for forceps in tedious labours. *Mon. J. med. Sci., 9,* 556.

1850. Some notes on the analogy between puerperal fever and surgical fever. *Mon. J. med. Sci., 2,* 414.

1851. On the communicability and propagation of puerperal fever. *Mon. J. med. Sci., 13,* 72.

1853. *Homoeopathy: its tenets and tendencies, Theoretical, Theo-*

logical and Therapeutical. Edinburgh.

1857. On ovariotomy and ovarian tapping. *Lancet, 1,* 285.

1859. Clinical lectures on the diseases of women. (The first of 38 lectures which embody Simpson's teaching at this time.) *Med. Times Gaz., 1,* 1.

1858. On the use of metallic sutures and metallic ligatures in surgical wounds and operations. *Med. Times Gaz., 1,* 571.

1859. Acupressure—a new method of arresting surgical haemorrhage. *Edinb. med. J., 5,* 645.

1860. On acupressure in amputation. *Med. Times Gaz., 1,* 137.

1860. On ovariotomy. *Med. Times. Gaz., 1,* 207.

1864. *Acupressure: a new method of arresting surgical haemorrhage and of accelerating the healing of wounds.* Edinburgh.

1867. Carbolic acid and its compounds in surgery. *Lancet, 2,* 546.

1868. Proposal to stamp out small pox. *Med. Times Gaz., 1,* 6.

1868. Our existing system of hospitalism and its effects. *Edinb. med. J., 14,* 816.

1869. Effects of hospitalism upon the mortality of limb amputations etc. *Bri. med. J., 1,* 93.

1869. A lecture on the Siamese and other united and viable twins. *Bri. med. J., 1,* 139.

Papers on Archaeological Subjects

From *Archaeological Essays by the late Sir James Young Simpson,* ed. by John Stuart, 1872, Edinburgh. The majority of these papers were published in the Edinburgh journals or as pamphlets.

1841. On leprosy and leper hospitals.

1851. Notices of ancient Roman medicine stamps etc. found in Great Britain.

1852. Notes on some ancient Greek medical vases for containing lykion: and on the modern use of the same drug in India.

1856. Was the Roman army provided with medical officers?

1857. On an old stone-roofed cell or oratory in the Island of Inchcolm.

1860. Archaeology: its past and its future work.

1861. On the Cat Stane, Kirkliston.

1861. On some Scottish magical charm stones or curing stones.

1862. Antiquarian notices of syphilis in Scotland.

1868. Is the Great Pyramid of Gizeh a metrological monument?

General Sources, References and Notes

A full search has been made in the contemporary medical journals for articles and letters written by Simpson and Syme. These journals are full of news items, gossip and often slander concerning the better known doctors of the time and Simpson and Syme feature prominently. While some other more obscure journals have been searched, the following have been most rewarding:

> *Association Medical Journal* (1853-1856).
> *British Medical Journal* (1857-1870).
> *Edinburgh Medical and Surgical Journal* (1805-1853).
> *Edinburgh Medical Journal* (1854-1870).
> *Lancet* (1823-1870).
> *Medical Times* (1842-1851).
> *Medical Times and Gazette* (1852-1870).
> *Monthly Journal of Medical Science* (1841-1855).
> *Provincial Medical and Surgical Journal* (1840-1852).

In the text the dates of the birth and death are given for most medical men mentioned. From the date of death it is a simple matter to trace an obituary notice in the *Lancet* or the *British Medical Journal*. In addition bibliographical material of some contemporary figures has been obtained from Plarr's *Lives of the Fellows of the Royal College of Surgeons of England* and from the *Dictionary of National Biography*.

Note: For each chapter a general source list is given followed by references and notes as numbered in the text. The sources of all quotations which appear in small print in the text are given in the reference list. Two major sources of references are abbreviated:

Mss RCS: Letters or documents in the Library of the Royal College of Surgeons, Edinburgh.

Mss EU: Letters or documents in the Library of Edinburgh University.

261

CHAPTER 1

General Sources

CHRISTISON, R. (1855). *Life of Sir Robert Christison Bart.* (Two volumes) London. The first volume is autobiographical and the second is edited by Christison's son. Both volumes give much detail of the medical scene in Edinburgh and there are many references to Syme and Simpson.

COCKBURN, H. (1913). *Memorials of his Time.* Edinburgh: Foulis. Published originally in 1865 these reminiscences of the well known legal luminary of Edinburgh provide a vivid picture of social life.

COMRIE, J. H. (1932). *History of Scottish Medicine.* London: Baillère, Tindall and Cox (Wellcome publication). This remarkable work in two volumes is quite indispensable to any student of medical history and, in particular, gives full and accurate information of every Edinburgh graduate of any distinction.

GRANT, A. (1884). *Story of the University of Edinburgh.* London: Blackwood.

GRAY, J. (1952). *History of Royal Medical Society.* Edinburgh: University Press.

GUTHRIE, D. (1963). *Janus in the Doorway.* London: Pitman. In this collection of essays on medical history there is much about the Edinburgh medical school.

HORN, D. B. (1967). *A Short History of the University of Edinburgh.* Edinburgh: University Press.

LONSDALE, H. (1870). *A Sketch of the Life and Writings of Robert Knox, the Anatomist.* London.

MASSON, D. (1892). *Edinburgh Sketches and Memories.* Edinburgh.

MILES, A. (1918). *The Edinburgh School of Surgery before Lister.* London.

WATT, F. (1913). *The Book of Edinburgh Anecdotes.* Edinburgh.

References and Notes

1. YOUNGSON, A. J. (1966). *The Making of Classical Edinburgh.* Edinburgh: University Press.
2. For the early history of the College of Surgeons see *History of the Royal College of Surgeons of Edinburgh*, by C. H. CRESSWELL published in Edinburgh in 1926 and an article by GAIRDNER (*Edinb. med. J.* 1859, 5, 789).
3. WRIGHT ST. CLAIR, R. E. (1964). *Doctors Monro—A Medical*

Saga. London: Wellcome Historical Medical Library.

4. GUTHRIE, D. (1965). *Extramural Education in Edinburgh*. Edinburgh: Livingstone.

5. Professor Alexander Simpson gives a full account of the history of the teaching of obstetrics in Edinburgh (*Edinb. med. J.* 1882, *28*, 481) and J. D. YOUNG writes about James Hamilton (*Med. Hist.* 1963, 7, 62).

6. TURNER, A. L. (1937). *Story of a Great Hospital. The Royal Infirmary of Edinburgh (1729-1929)*. Edinburgh: Oliver and Boyd.

7. The Edinburgh Infirmary nurses are referred to in *Lord Lister* by R. GODLEE, published in 1917 in London by Macmillan and in *Lord Lister* by D. GUTHRIE, published in 1948 in Edinburgh by Livingstone.

8. BROCK, LORD (1952). *The Life and Work of Astley Cooper*. Edinburgh: Livingstone.

9. Mss RCS.

CHAPTER 2

General Sources

Much information in this chapter is derived from Paterson (see Biographical Sources) and from Christison (see General Sources to Chap. 1). Details of the Syme family have been checked in the Signet Library, Edinburgh.

References and Notes

10. ROBERTSON, D. (1935). *The Princes Street Proprietors and other Chapters in the History of the Royal Burgh of Edinburgh*. Edinburgh: Oliver and Boyd.

11. Register Office, Edinburgh.

12. ANNALS OF PHILOSOPHY, 1818.

13. EDINBURGH MEDICAL AND SURGICAL JOURNAL (1824), *21*, 19.

14. PATERSON, R. (1874). *Memorials of the Life of James Syme* Edinburgh: Edmonston and Douglas.

15. Dr Scott was probably a physician who studied in Paris under Laennec and introduced the stethoscope to Edinburgh. While Paterson gives some details of Syme's continental tour there are no other records, except a casual mention in Syme's later writings of his admiration for the work of Professor Rust, a Berlin surgeon.

16. CROSSE, V. M. (1968). *A Surgeon in the Early Nineteenth Century. The Life and Times of John Green Crosse*. Edinburgh: Livingstone.

17. PEDDIE, A. *Dr John Brown: his Life and Work. With Narrative Sketches of James Syme.* Harveian Festival Oration in 1890. Reprinted as a pamphlet from *Edinburgh Medical Journal.*

18. MEDICAL TIMES (1844). *11*, 23. (Simpson escaped attention in this satiric series.)

<h2 align="center">CHAPTER 3</h2>

General Sources

The biographies by Duns and Eve Simpson have been drawn upon for this chapter and details have been checked from papers in the RCS Mss. Reference has been made to Burke's Peerage for the Simpson lineage. Mr John Simpson has given me a family tree which is continued to the present day.

References and Notes

19. Register Office, Edinburgh.

20. It has frequently been stated that Simpson was born in the house shown to the right of Plate 1. Eve Simpson, however, wrote in 1911 (*Edinb. med. J.*, 1911, *6*, 482.) 'The house at Bathgate in which James Simpson was born . . . is now a mission hall, bought and given to his native town by a grateful patient in his memory . . . the house opposite is the one he was brought up in, for his father, the baker's fortune improving, they moved across the way.'

Main Street, at its lower end, is now dilapidated. The houses shown in the right of the Plate have been demolished. If Eve's description is correct (and it seems likely to be so) the birthplace was demolished early in 1969. It had stood neglected and a mere shell but identified by a plaque which described its use as a mission hall. Perhaps it was too late to preserve it but I cannot fail to contrast the devoted care given to the restoration of the house of Ephraim MacDowell, the pioneer ovariotomist, in Danville, Kentucky. It is to be hoped that local and national pride will yet combine to mark the site of Simpson's birthplace in some appropriate way.

21. WILSON, A. (1852). *Life of Dr John Reid.* Edinburgh.

22. The diary mentioned has not been traced but Duns apparently saw it.

23. Simpson's class tickets can be seen in the Edinburgh University Library and there is a certificate from Pillans, Professor of Humanity, who writes of his pupil: 'attended class 1825-26 with great regularity, that his general conduct was

exemplary and that his appearances and exercises give distinguished proof of diligence and proficiency in his studies.' In Mss RCS there are a few papers from his student days and we find that Lizars' anatomy course cost £3 3s., Monro's anatomy course £4 4s. and Graham's botany course £4 9s.

24. Mss RCS.
25. Mss RCS.
26. Mss RCS.
27. I have not been able to trace the journal which Simpson kept on his continental tour and to which Duns refers. There are some details of the trip in letters in the separate collection in the RCS.
28. Mss RCS.
29. Mss RCS.
30. This description of Simpson is from an obituary notice in *The Scotsman* of 1870.

CHAPTER 4

General Sources

Some sources listed for Chapter 1 have been of particular value for this chapter. Much has been taken from the biographies. The records of the College of Surgeons and the University of Edinburgh have been examined.

References and Notes

31. Dr Brown's series of essays *Horae Subsecivae* first appeared in 1858 and ran to many editions. *Rab and His Friends* was first published in 1859.
32. *Letters of Dr John Brown.* Edited by his son and by D. W. Forrest and published in 1907 in London by Black.
33. When Syme read his first communication to the Royal Medical Society about 1820 this was reported as 'objectionable on account of the asperity of censure and personality of allusion in which it indulged'. (Gray, J., 1952. *History of Royal Medical Society.* Edinburgh: University Press.)
34. Minutes of Royal College of Surgeons of Edinburgh for 1832.
35. Lizars was for several years in the Navy before settling down in Edinburgh and his service career can be traced in the Public Records Office. Like Syme he was subjected to a caricature in the *Medical Times* (1845, *112*, 47). His obituary notices do him scant justice but he received some attention on the anniversary of his death (*Br. med. J.*, 1960, 2, 1665).

For his work on ovariotomy see *Spencer Wells* by J. A. Shepherd, published in 1965 in Edinburgh by Livingstone.

36. Copies of Syme's original and renewed Commissions are in Mss RCS and in the Wellcome Library respectively.
37. The originals of Simpson's testimonials are in Mss RCS. A printed copy is in the Library of the Royal College of Physicians of Edinburgh.
38. Mss RCS.
39. Mss RCS.
40. There is a printed copy of the catalogue of Simpson's Museum in the Edinburgh University Library.
41. Mss RCS.
42. Mss RCS.
43. Syme's opinion is quoted in Paterson (see ref. 14).

CHAPTER 5

General Sources

The events recorded in the chapter are fully reported in the medical journals. Various pamphlets and other documents which have been consulted are mostly in Mss RCS.

References and Notes

44. LIZARS, J. (1838). *System of Practical Surgery*, Edinburgh.
45. Full accounts of Syme *v.* Lizars were published in pamphlets in 1840 and in contemporary journals (e.g. *Lancet*, 1840, 2, 202).
46. Two important pamphlets are *Statement by Dr Christison and Professor Syme with concurrence of other members of the Medical Faculty as to the Suppression of the Chair of General Pathology* (1841) and *Memorial on the Propriety of continuing the Chair of General Pathology* by J. Y. Simpson (1841).
47. Mss RCS.
48. Mss RCS.
49. BRITISH AND FOREIGN MEDICO-CHIRURGICAL REVIEW (1848). 2, 31.
50. GUTHRIE, D. (1948). *Lord Lister*, Edinburgh: Livingstone.
51. LANCET (1865). *1*, 333.
52. CHALMERS, J. A. (1963). *J. Obstet. Gynaec. Br. Commonw.* 70, 94. A review of the story of the suction tractor.
53. MOIR, J. C. (1949). *Br. med. J., 1*, 69. A discussion of Simpson's article.
54. The amputation statistics collected by Simpson are in Mss

RCS and the documents are signed by well known surgeons in many instances.

55. WILLIAMS, L. (1963). *J. Obstet. Gynaec. Br. Commonw.* 70, 167. Simpson's teaching methods are referred to in detail.

56. Mss EU.

57. DUNS, J. (1873). *Memoir of Sir James Y. Simpson.* Edinburgh: Edmonston and Douglas.

58. GORDON-TAYLOR, G., & WALLS, E. W. (1958). *Sir Charles Bell. His Life and Times.* Edinburgh: Livingstone.

59. CHRISTISON, R. (1885). *Life of Sir Robert Christison Bart.* London.

60. PATERSON (see ref. 14).

61. The U.C.H. affair is reported in great detail in all the medical journals. For the quarrel with Liston see in particular *Mon. J. med. Sci.* (1846), 6, 67.

62. *Letters of Dr John Brown* (see ref. 32).

CHAPTER 6

General Sources

Of many volumes devoted primarily to the history of anaesthesia the following have been particularly useful:

DUNCUM, A. B. M. (1947). *The Development of Inhalation Anaesthesia.* London: Wellcome Publication.

KEYS, T. E. (1963). *The History of Surgical Anaesthesia,* 2nd ed. New York: Schuman.

SYKES, W. S. (1961). *Essays on the First Hundred Years of Anaesthesia,* (2 vols). Edinburgh: Livingstone.

Of countless papers those listed below have special reference to Edinburgh events:

MILLER, J. (1848). *Surgical Experience of Chloroform.* (Pamphlet.)

BRITISH MEDICAL JOURNAL (1896). Jubilee of anaesthesia. *Br. med. J.*, 2, 1135.

EDINBURGH MEDICAL JOURNAL (1911). Jubilee of birth of Simpson. *Edinb. med. J.*, 6, 481.

CLARK, A. J. (1938). Aspects of the history of anaesthesia. *Br. med. J.*, 2, 1029.

JOHNSTONE, R. W. (1947). James Young Simpson and chloroform. *Edinb. med. J.*, 54, 324.

MOIR, J. C. (1947). November 1847 and its sequel. *Edinb. med. J.*, 54, 593.

MOIR, J. C. (1948). A note on the centenary of chloroform. *Proc. R. Soc. Med.*, 41, 28.

HOVELL, B. C., & WILSON, J. (1969). The history of anaesthesia in
Edinburgh. *J. R. Coll. Surg. Edinb., 14,* 107.

Nearly every number of the medical journals in the years after
1847 has some reference to anaesthesia. These must be read to
grasp the impact of the new discovery, to appreciate the rapidity
with which both ether and chloroform were taken up throughout
the world and to sense the rivalries and the controversies.

References and Notes

63. CARTWRIGHT, F. F. (1952). *The English Pioneers of Anaesthesia (Beddoes: Davy: Hickman).* Bristol: Wright.

64. The relative claims for priority by Wells and Morton are
discussed at great length in all the histories of anaesthesia
and were the subject even of government reports in the
U.S.A. Long's claims are dealt with in the *Bulletin of the
History Medicine* (1943) *13,* 340.

65. For accounts of Liston's operation see:
SQUIRE, W. (1888). *Lancet,* 2, 1220.
COCK, F. W. (1915). *Am. J. Surg.* 29, 98.
BRITISH MEDICAL JOURNAL (1896). 2, 1135.

66. In an address at Liverpool in 1896 Lister stated 'I witnessed
the first operation in England under ether, it was performed
by Robert Liston. . . . Soon afterwards I saw the same great
surgeon amputate the thigh, by aid of another agent chloroform . . .' (*Collected Papers of Joseph, Baron Lister,* vol. 2,
1909). This is the only suggestion I can trace of Lister's
presence at Liston's first major operation under ether. When
Lister said this he was aged 70 and his memory may have
played him false. There must have been nearly a year
between Liston's first use of ether and his first use of chloroform. If he did use chloroform this must have been in late
November 1847. Liston was ill from August to November
1847 but returned to work briefly about 28th November.
He died on 12th December. The *Medical Times* of December 4th reported that Liston, amongst other London surgeons
had used chloroform. It seems likely that a thigh amputation
with a new anaesthetic would have been mentioned specifi-
cally. No record of such an operation can be traced in
the U.C.H. operating lists. Lister's statement may be inaccurate although he must have heard of Liston's first use of
ether and would certainly have seen many later operations
under ether or chloroform.

67. Simpson was accustomed to mention the Dumfries operation in his lectures. The event has been investigated by

T. W. Bailie (*Br. J. of Anaesth.* 1965, *37*, 952). The same writer has a short monograph *From Boston to Dumfries* published in 1966 for private circulation in Dumfries.

68. DEGENSHEIM, G. A. & HURWITZ, A. (1961). An intimate view of the Letheon controversy. *Surgery, 50,* 716.

69. MONTHLY JOURNAL OF MEDICAL SCIENCE (1849). *9,* 628.

70. ROBINSON, J. (1847). *A Treatise on the Inhalation of Ether for the Prevention of Pain in Surgical Operations: containing a Numerous Collection of Cases in which it has been applied.* (Robinson is described as 'Surgeon Dentist to the Metropolitan Hospital'.)

71. For an account of Mesmer see *Anton Mesmer* by D. M. Walmsley, published in 1967 in London by Hale. Esdaile published *Mesmerism in India and its Application in Surgery and Medicine* in 1846. Braid published *Neuropnology: or the rationale of nervous sleep* in 1843. Elliotson was ostracised by his colleagues for his publication of *Numerous cases of surgical operations without pain in the mesmeric state,* in 1843.

72. Simpson's references to his visit to Liston at the end of 1846 are very brief and appear late in his life in various published lectures.

73. NORTH BRITISH REVIEW (1847). *9,* 169.

74. Mss EU. But see also B. C. Hovell and J. Wilson who, in their survey of the history of anaesthesia in Edinburgh (*Jl R. Coll. Surg. Edinb.* 1969, *14,* 107), draw attention to a report in the *Edinburgh Evening Courant* of 14th January 1847. From this report it appears that the first major operation under ether anaesthesia in Edinburgh was performed by James Duncan, a senior surgeon in the Royal Infirmary, on January 9th, the procedure being a mid-thigh amputation.

75. MONTHLY JOURNAL OF MEDICAL SCIENCE (1847). *8,* 218. Syme wrote also 'Operations performed quickly are in general performed well, not because of the short time they occupy but in consequence of nothing more being done by them but what is actually required: while slow operations are in general ill-performed, not by reason of their slowness, but from the unnecessary groping, squeezing, cutting and teasing required for their completion. . . .' (*Mon. J. med. Sci.* 1847, *8,* 73).

76. Mss RCS.

77. MONTHLY JOURNAL OF MEDICAL SCIENCE (1847), *8,* 72.

78. Snow's opinions are to be found in the journals from 1848

to 1857 and in his posthumous publication *On chloroform and other anaesthetics* published in 1858 in which there is a short biography by Richardson. Snow refers to the 'slovenly and uncleanly manner' in which chloroform was given in Edinburgh. Snow and his London colleagues no doubt were somewhat tired of being told by Simpson that they did not know how to use chloroform!

79. All these returns are in Mss RCS.
80. Mss RCS.
81. SIMPSON, EVE (1896). *Sir James Y. Simpson*. New York: Scribner.
82. LANCET (1847). 2, 571. It is likely that Lawrence used a mixture of ether and chloroform or an impure chloroform. (See also *Med. Times Gaz.*, 1875, *1*, 586.)
83. A large dossier on the Waldie controversy is in the Library of the Liverpool Medical Institution. This includes the letters by Waldie and his brother which I quote. Amongst the pamphlets are Waldie's address to the Liverpool Philosophical Society in November 1847 and George Waldie's defence of his brother in 1870.

    Simpson's visit to Liverpool in 1847 is recorded in the Minutes of the Medical Institution.

    The following papers may be consulted about Waldie:
    DILLING, W. J. (1934). *Lpool med.-chir. J. 42*, 82
    O'LEARY, A. J. (1935). *Br. J. Anaesth. 12*, 41.
    DUNDEE, J. W. (1953). *Anaesthesia. 8*, 218.
84. LANCET (1870) 2, 16.
85. THORNTON, J. L. (1949). *The relationship between James Matthews Duncan and Sir James Young Simpson. Medicine Ill. 3*, 268.
    (See also the obituary of Duncan by W. Turner in *St Bart's Hosp. Rep.* 1890, *26*, 23.)
86. Mss RCS.
87. Eve Simpson (see ref. 81).
88. MONTHLY JOURNAL OF MEDICAL SCIENCE (1847). *8*, 415.
89. MITFORD, NANCY (1938). *The Ladies of Alderley*. London: Chapman and Hall. (Reprinted by permission of A. D. Peters & Company.)
90. GREAM, G. T. (1849). *The Misapplication of anaesthesia in Childbirth exemplified by Facts*. London. This is typical of many pamphlets against anaesthesia.
91. Mss RCS.
92. In the *Medical Times* (1848, *17*, 308) there is a note that the Court had left Windsor and that the *Edinburgh Witness* had

reported 'Professor Simpson would be required with his services and chloroform for the forthcoming confinement'. The report was denied by the *Caledonian Mercury*. Queen Victoria gave birth to a daughter, Princess Louise, that year. Had Simpson been called to Windsor for this occasion and had he used general anaesthesia successfully, public reaction would have been rapid and might have led to an earlier acceptance of general anaesthesia in childbirth.

93. Hannah Greener's death is very fully discussed in the journals (e.g. *Edinb. med. surg. J.* 1848, *69*, 498). W. S. Sykes analyses the case in his *First Hundred Years of Anaesthesia* published in Edinburgh in 1961 by Livingstone.

94. Sykes (see ref. 93) is rather hard on Simpson and his faulty statistics, forgetting that Simpson at least tried to use statistics intelligently while most medical men had no use for them at all!

95. The Bigelow correspondence appears in the journals of January 1870. One of Simpson's last literary efforts was a very fair account of the parts played by Morton and Wells (*Med. Times Gaz.* 1870, *1*, 90).

CHAPTER 7

General Sources

All the topics in this chapter are well covered in contemporary medical journals and in various monographs and pamphlets.

Sources of information about the medical aspects of the Crimean War abound, particularly in the biographies of Miss Nightingale. There are letters from Simpson concerning the war in Mss RCS, in the Bowman collection (see reference 107) and in the Library of the RAMC at Millbank.

There is a great deal of information about homoeopathy in Simpson's book *Homoeopathy. Its tenets and tendencies, theoretical, theological and therapeutical*. This was published in 1853 as the 'third edition'. Previous editions were shorter and in pamphlet form.

The subject of medical reform fills the medical journals of the day and is well covered in McMenemy's life of Charles Hastings (see reference 102).

References and Notes

96. JAMESON, E. (1961). *Natural History of Quackery*. London: Joseph.

97. MEDICAL TIMES (1845). *13*, 21.

98. Henderson's pamphlets *An Enquiry into the Homoeopathic Practice of Medicine* (1845) and *Reply to Dr Simpson's Pamphlet on Homoeopathy* (1852) are typical of many on the subject.

99. The proceedings of the society are reported fully in the *Monthly Journal of Medical Science* (1851), *13*, 581.

100. Simpson's volume on homoeopathy (see above).

101. Mss RCS.

102. McMenemy, W. H. (1959). *The Life and Times of Sir Charles Hastings*. Edinburgh: Livingstone.

103. Christison (see ref. 59).

104. Mss RAMC Library, Millbank.

105. *Illustrated London News*, September 23rd, 1854.

106. *The Times*, October 12th, 1854.

107. Thomas, K. B. (1966). The manuscripts of Sir William Bowman. *Med. Hist. 10*, 252.

108. Manuscript in private ownership.

109. Manuscript in private ownership.

110. Shepherd, J. A. (1966). The civil hospitals in the Crimea 1855-1856. *Proc. R. Soc. Med. 59*, 199.

111. Cope, Z. (1965). Extracts from the diary of Thomas Laycock. *Med Hist. 9*, 169.

112. Monthly Journal of Medical Science (1852). 2, 284.

113. Edinburgh Medical Journal (1855). *1*, 224.

114. Monthly Journal of Medical Science (1852). *15*, 274.

115. Lancet (1850). *1*, 605.

116. Monthly Journal of Medical Science (1851). *13*, 198.

117. The litigation is reported in the *Monthly Journal of Medical Science* (1852), *15*, 182.

118. The litigation is reported in the *Lancet* (1855). *1*, 103.

119. Medical Times and Gazette (1857). *1*, 632.

120. This and the three following quotations are from *Stories of the Temple in Edinburgh* by 'An Acolyte', published in London by Vickers in 1862. The book was almost certainly suppressed. I have traced four copies: in the British Museum, the Royal College of Surgeons of Edinburgh, the Glasgow University Library and the Edinburgh City Library. A pencil note in the latter copy suggests that Syme wrote this book but this is very unlikely as the style is not his. No doubt he took a sardonic pleasure in reading it, if a copy came his way!

121. Mss RCS.

CHAPTER 8

General Sources
   Much more can be learnt of the private life of Simpson than
that of Syme. This is mainly because of the large volume of
private papers which survive relating to the former.

References and Notes
122. MONTHLY JOURNAL OF MEDICAL SCIENCE (1851). 2, 53.
123. *Letters of Dr John Brown* (see ref. 32).
124. GODLEE, R. J. (1917). *Lord Lister.* London: Macmillan.
125. GODLEE, R. J. (1917). *Lord Lister.* London: Macmillan.
126. The Queen Street house survives with its exterior relatively
     unaltered but for a plaque to record Simpson's occupancy.
     Some of the original furniture is retained in the dining room
     where the chloroform experiments were done but the rest
     of the house is used for offices and is now somewhat neglec-
     ted.
127. Storer sent his reminiscences to Sir Alexander Simpson
     and they were published in the *Edinburgh Medical Journal*
     (1911), 7, 12.
128. Mss RCS.
129. LUTYENS, M. (1965). *Effie in Venice.* London: Murray.
130. LUTYENS, M. (1967). *Millais and the Ruskins.* London:
     Murray.
131. Simpson gives a full account of oil inunction in a pamphlet
     (reprinted from *Mon. J. med. Sci.* 1853, *15*, 316).
132. Mss RCS.
133. *Medical Times and Gazette* (1858). 2, 65.
134. Eve Simpson (see ref. 81).
135. Spencer Wells gave this account when he paid a tribute on
     Simpson's death (*Br. med. J.* 1870, 2, 52).
136. LONSDALE, H. (1870). *A Sketch of the Life and Writings of
     Robert Knox, the Anatomist.* London.
137. Mss RCS.
138. Viewbank is still occupied and is a charming house in a
     secluded garden just to the West of Granton in Laverock
     Road. The original simple square building faces south and
     a more ornate extension was built by Simpson and overlooks
     the Firth of Forth and the Fife hills. In the garden there is
     a statue of one of Simpson's favourite dogs.
139. There are two full biographies of Lawson Tait:
     MCKAY, W. J. S. (1922). *Lawson Tait. His Life and Work.*

London: Bailliere, Tindall & Cox.

FLACK, I. H. (1949). *Lawson Tait*. London: Heinemann.
140. WILSON (see ref. 21).
141. Mss RCS.
142. SHEPHERD, J. A. (1965). *Spencer Wells*. Edinburgh: Livingstone.
143. Mss RCS.
144. Mss RCS.
145. Simpson's archaeological writings are given under Selected Writings of Simpson (p. 260) and were collected and edited by John Stuart in 1872 under the title *Archaeological Essays by the late Sir James Young Simpson*.
146. Mss RCS.
147. Mss RCS.
148. For an account of Simpson's library see:
GUNN, A. (1968). *J. Obstet. Gynaec. Br. Commonw.* 15, 249. I have in my possession *De Recta Curandorum Vulnerum* by Franciscus Arcaeus published in Amsterdam in 1658 and bearing Simpson's signature. I am fortunate to have acquired this very rare volume once owned by Simpson. It was given to me by my father, the late F. P. Shepherd, M.A., F.E.I.S., who, being a classical scholar, often picked up such items in the Edinburgh bookstalls. This rarity he acquired for a shilling about 1910 and its possession by Simpson indicates the latter's antiquarian tastes.
149. The Disruption was on May 18th, 1843. The separatists left the Assembly at St Andrew's Church and marched to a warehouse in Tanfield where a large congregation was already installed and all preparations had been made for a ceremony to establish a Free Church. Simpson may have marched to Tanfield but it is more likely that he was already in his seat awaiting the rebels. Professor Miller was also there and both he and Simpson are depicted in D. O. Hill's painting of the historic scene (Plate 15). The Rev. Thomas Brown gives a full account of the occasion in his *Annals of the Disruption* (1893) and mentions Simpson as a prominent layman who supported the movement.
150. Mss RCS.
151. This and the four following letters quoted are in Mss RCS with many other documents concerning the Q. family. There are also various receipts for payments to foster parents for other infants placed by Simpson. Simpson's original letters are not extant but there are many copies or rough drafts of his replies to the persistent Mrs Q. The ultimate fate of

Mr and Mrs Q. and their adopted child has not been traced. The child may have survived to adult life and established a family and for this reason the surname has been withheld.

CHAPTER 9

General Sources

Until 1869 acupressure was discussed very fully in the medical journals. Much of Simpson's large correspondence on the subject still survives.

Ovariotomy was the subject of much argument from about 1840 to 1865. For a history of ovariotomy the reader is referred to Chapter 4 of the writer's life of Spencer Wells (see ref. 142). Letters between Spencer Wells and Simpson on the subject of ovariotomy are in Mss RCS.

References and Notes

152. LANCET (1862). *1*, 203.
153. CHRISTISON (see ref. 59).
154. John Bell's description is quoted by Simpson in *Acupressure: a new method of arresting haemorrhage and of accelerating the healing of wounds* published in Edinburgh in 1864.
155. Paré is quoted freely in Simpson's book (see ref. 154).
156. See Simpson's book on acupressure (ref. 154).
157. This address is printed in a pamphlet (undated).
158. Simpson described his first animal experiments to the Medico-chirurgical Society in October 1858. (*Edinb. med. J.* 1858, *4*, 547.) He gave a report on his technique to the Royal Society of Edinburgh on December 9th, 1858 (*Edinb. med. J.* 1859, *5*, 645). For the next few years he kept up a constant flow of observations from his own experience or from that of others. He delighted in placing Shakespearean quotations at the head of these articles such as 'Come lay aside your stitching'.
159. From Simpson's book of acupressure (see ref. 154).
160. TAIT, L. (1865). Acupressure: experiments on the lower animals. *Med. Times Gaz. 1*, 502. (In later life Tait became an ardent antivivisectionist!)
161. Mss RCS.
162. Mss RCS.
163. Mss RCS.
164. Mss RCS.
165. Mss RCS.
166. Mss RCS.

167. Mss RCS.
168. The 'execution' of Simpson's pamphlet was described with some relish in the contemporary journals (e.g. *Med. Times Gaz.* 1865, *1*, 236). Prolonged and bitter arguments continued in the correspondence columns of the *Lancet* and the *Medical Times and Gazette* for a whole year.
169. BRITISH MEDICAL JOURNAL (1865). 2, 691.
170. The medical historian sometimes has the opportunity of testing methods which have been advocated in the past and then discarded. I have done this to a limited extent for acupressure. Large blood-vessels just under the skin (e.g. in amputation flaps) are readily controlled by Simpson's first method of acupressure. Major arteries divided at amputation are not so easily controlled in this way. The more elaborate methods with wire loops have not been tried but would, I believe, be safe. I have tried Simpson's method of controlling the ovarian pedicle with acupressure but found that the thin stretched muscles of the abdominal wall offer a poor counter against which to exert pressure. I should mention that I have only experimented with the *temporary* control of blood vessels and have hardly felt justified in sending a patient back to the ward impaled with needles or pins for permanent haemostasis! Nevertheless my impression is that in many situations acupressure does all that Simpson claimed for it.
171. This letter is in the Library of the Royal College of Surgeons of England.
172. McDowell's cases were published in an obscure American journal and there were disbelieving comments in the British press. Lizars published his cases in 1825 in a large folio, with coloured plates: *On the extirpation of Diseased Ovaria*.
173. Clay's cases are recorded from 1842 onwards in the *Medical Times*.
174. Handyside's operation is reported in the *Edinburgh Medical Journal* (1846, *65*, 279) and the discussion which followed in the *Monthly Journal of Medical Science* (1846, *6*, 53).
175. Clay's visit is recorded in the *Monthly Journal of Medical Science* (1848, *8*, 761).
176. Edward's operation is reported in the *Edinburgh Medical Journal* (1856, *2*, 752). Not much is known of Edwards except that he came to Edinburgh from Kings College Hospital where he had worked with Fergusson. A promising career seems to have been cut short by illness.
177. Mss RCS.

178. Mss RCS.
179. Mss EU.
180. Mss RCS.
181. Mss RCS.
182. Mss RCS.
183. BRITISH MEDICAL JOURNAL (1865). 2, 142.
184. The Alloa case is reported in the *British Medical Journal* (1870, *1*, 159). This is one of the last of Simpson's clinical writings.
185. Professor Courty's *Excursion Chirurgicale en Angleterre* was published in 1863. A copy of this rare book is in the Library of the Royal College of Surgeons of England. The dedication to Simpson reads 'en memoire de l'appui que l'autorité de votre parole a donné depuis longtemps a l'ovariotomie'. Courty states that he saw Simpson do a successful ovariotomy in 1863 and that this was Simpson's first attempt at the operation.

CHAPTER 10

General Sources

A full bibliography concerning Lister and his ideas is not considered necessary. Godlee's *Life of Lister* remains an invaluable account. There are modern assessments of Lister in a special number of the *British Journal of Surgery* in 1967 to mark the centenary of the publication of the antiseptic system. Of particular value is the paper by F. N. L. Poynter, 'The Contemporary Scientific background of Lister's achievement' and I have quoted from this in the first paragraph of this chapter.

Simpson's work on hospitalism is recorded in detail in the medical journals and there is a useful assessment by S. Selwyn, 'Sir James Simpson and Hospital Cross-Infection' in *Medical History* (1965, *10*, 241).

References and Notes

186. Much has been written about Semmelweiss including a biography:
SINCLAIR, W. J. (1909). *Semmelweiss: His Life and Doctrine.* Manchester.
Two papers given on the centenary of his death are useful summaries (*Proc. R. Soc. Med.* 1966, *59*, 29).
187. Routh's paper is reported in *Medico-Chirurgical Transactions* (1849, *32*, 27) and Arneth's paper in the *Monthly Journal of Medical Science* (1851, *12*, 505).

188. MONTHLY JOURNAL OF MEDICAL SCIENCE (1849). *9*, 329.
189. MONTHLY JOURNAL OF MEDICAL SCIENCE (1850). *10*, 414.
190. From a lecture 'Surgical Fevers' in the *Medical Times and Gazette* (1859, *1*, 411).
191. From a lecture 'Surgical Fevers' in the *Medical Times and Gazette* (1859, *1*, 411).
192. HOLMES, T. (1860). *A System of Surgery*. London.
193. FERGUSSON, A. (1870). *A System of Practical Surgery*. London.
194. SIMPSON, D. C. & WALLACE, A. B. (1956). Edinburgh's first burn hospital. *Jl R. Coll. Surg. Edinb.* 2, 134.
195. LANCET (1867). 2, 246.
196. The paper by Hughes Bennet is in the *Edinburgh Medical Journal* (1867, *13*, 810). Calvert's paper is in the *Lancet* 1863, 2, 362). D. C. Schechter and H. Swan in 'Jules Lemaire: a forgotten hero of surgery' (*Surgery*, 1961, *49*, 817) discuss Lemaire's part in the evolution of the use of carbolic acid.
197. Smith's paper is reported in the *British Medical Journal* (1867). 2, 121.
198. Pirrie's paper is reported in the *British Medical Journal* (1867). 2, 171 and Lister's paper was published later in the *British Medical Journal* (1867) 2, 246.
199. LANCET (1867), 2, 546.
200. LANCET (1867). 2, 595.
201. Manuscript in the Wellcome Collection.
202. BRITISH MEDICAL JOURNAL (1869). 2, 107.
203. MEDICAL TIMES AND GAZETTE (1869). 2, 265.
204. There is a copy of Dr Parkes' report on the hospital in Renkioi in the RAMC Library, Millbank. See also:
   SHEPHERD, J. A. (1966). The civil hospitals in the Crimea 1855-1856. *Proc. R. Soc. Med.* 59, 199.
205. Simpson's articles on hospitalism appear in many periodicals but the fullest texts are in the *Edinburgh Medical Journal* (1868, *14*, 816).
206. LANCET (1869). 2, 194.
207. LANCET (1869). 2, 451.
208. BRITISH MEDICAL JOURNAL (1868). *1*, 1.
209. Manuscript in the Lister Collection of the Royal College of Surgeons of England.

GENERAL SOURCES, REFERENCES AND NOTES

CHAPTER 11

General Sources

This account of the last years of Syme and Simpson is derived largely from the biographies. The final illnesses of both men were followed closely in the medical journals.

The election to the Principalship of Edinburgh University attracted much interest in the lay and medical press. Duns covers this subject incompletely and the official university records are silent. There are details of the background of such elections in Christison's life. My reconstruction of this cause célèbre is made from the large collection of manuscript documents in the Royal College of Surgeons of Edinburgh. There are many originals of letters on the controversy and many drafts in Simpson's hand. There are two printed documents of special value. The first is *Principalship of the University*, a privately printed sheet in support of Grant. The second is *Principalship of the University of Edinburgh* published as a pamphlet in October 1868, by Simpson's supporters. There may well have been other such pamphlets from both factions.

References and Notes

210. The medical journals of 1869 have many references to the tour of the Siamese twins in Europe. Simpson's account is in the *British Medical Journal* (1869, *1*, 139).

211. Simpson's earliest experimental work is described by Henry Imlach, 'Observations and Experiments in softening, erosion and perforation of the stomach' in the *Edinburgh Medical Journal* (1837, 47, 391). Eve Simpson gives anecdotes and descriptions of the family dogs in her biography and in a small monograph.

212. COPE, Z. (1965). Extracts from the diary of Thomas Laycock. *Med. Hist.* 9, 169.

213. MANTON, J. (1965). *Elizabeth Garret Anderson*. London: Methuen.

214. Details of Brewster are to be found in Grant's *Story of the University of Edinburgh* (London: Blackwood. 1884) and in *Dictionary of National Biography*.

215. *Dictionary of National Biography*.

216. Mss RCS.

217. Mss RCS.

218. Mss RCS. (The identity of the Rev. Blackie is uncertain. He is referred to in the documents variously as Professor,

279

Rev. or Dr Blackie. His signature to some letters is W. A. Blackie. He was not, therefore, the better known Stuart Blackie, Professor of Greek, a man of wit and some notoriety.)

219. Mss RCS.
220. Mss RCS.
221. Mss RCS.
222. Mss RCS.
223. Mss RCS. (It must be admitted that the only copy available of this statement is in Simpson's hand: it is at least possible that he composed it and *hoped* that the Colleges would support it!)
224. Mss RCS. (There are many such rough drafts and perhaps some pamphlets were printed and circulated in Simpson's defence; certainly these rather pathetic notes formed the substance of many letters to his friends.)
225. There is an obituary of David Simpson in the *Edinburgh Medical Journal* (1865, *11*, 773). Simpson enjoyed choosing his coat of arms and the motto *Victor dolore*. It is no doubt apocryphal that a friend suggested that a new born baby should be a central feature with the motto 'Does your mother know you are out?' for this smacks of a humour of a later date!
226. Mss RCS.
227. Lancet (1866). *1*, 578.
228. Lister's selection was deplored in some quarters. The *Medical Times and Gazette* (1869, 2, 109) saw no reason why an Englishman should be elected and hinted at nepotism on Syme's part. It was stated too that Lister's work had not been in practical surgery and that carbolic was the invention of a Frenchman and of doubtful value!

The quarrel with Spence is recorded in a paper by H. A. F. Dudley and D. Simpson, entitled 'A surgical contretemps of 1869 and its effects' (*Jl. R. Coll. Surg. Edinb.* 1964, *10*, 72).
229. Edinburgh Medical Journal (1868). *14*, 199.
230. Simpson gave evidence in London in the Mordaunt divorce case in which the Prince of Wales was indirectly involved. The complicated medical aspects of this case are summarised in the *Medical Times and Gazette* (1870, *1*, 270).
231. Probably at Simpson's own request an autopsy was performed. As customary the report was given full publicity. A great deal of attention was paid to the brain and although the weight of this organ (then thought to have some relation to intellect) did not equal that of other great men

'the convolutions of the cerebrum were remarkable, for their number, depth and the intricate nature of their foldings' (*Lancet*, 1870, *1*, 717). It was believed that mental vigour depended on the extent of the convolutions and Simpson's brain presented 'an appearance not soon to be forgotten by those privileged to see it in the apparently increased number of convolutions and their great size and development'. The heart was the seat of gross disease with valvular lesions, fatty degeneration and an aneurysm on the wall of the right ventricle.

CHAPTER 12

General Sources
Contemporary assessments of Syme and Simpson are to be found in the obituaries in the medical journals and the Edinburgh newspapers. Much more has been written about Simpson than about Syme in succeeding years.

References and Notes
232. Mss RCS.
233. Simpson, his wife and children are buried in Warriston Cemetery on a small mound, dominated by an obelisk.
234. There are portraits of Simpson in oil and many photographs, engravings and prints. A notable painting is one by Macbeth in the Royal College of Physicians of Edinburgh.
235. Details of Walter Simpson may be found in biographies of R. L. Stevenson.
236. Alexander Simpson's stormy inaugural lecture is reported in the *British Medical Journal* (1870, 2, 515). When he was made professor there was a protest meeting even in London. When he died in 1916, tribute was made to his 'benificent and benevolent domination' and to his part in developing operative gynaecology. He shared his uncle's tendency for evangelistic activities. He was apprenticed to the anatomist Goodsir and was a dresser to Syme as a student.
237. It has been recorded that Mrs Simpson poured out more tea than anyone in Scotland!
238. Syme's grave is marked by a simple memorial slab set in a low wall in the East graveyard of St John's Church, Princes Street.
239. Of notable oil paintings of Syme one by George Richmond is in the Scottish National Portrait Gallery and was probably painted about 1855. Another hangs in the Royal College

of Surgeons of Edinburgh and was painted by an unknown artist about 1865.

240. Brown's letter is in the Lister Collection in the Royal College of Surgeons of England.

241. Godlee's life of Lister (see ref. 125).

242. Of many assessments of Simpson's work in obstetrics and gynaecology may be mentioned those by F. W. N. Haultain (*Edinb. med. J.* 1911, *6*, 505) and by A. L. Gunn (*J. Obstet. Gynaec. Br. Commonw.* 1968, *3*, 249).

Index of Names

INDEX OF NAMES

General Index

PRINTED IN GREAT BRITAIN BY
NORTHUMBERLAND PRESS LIMITED
GATESHEAD